RENAL DIET COOKBOOK FOR BEGINNERS

The Essential Renal Diet Guide
to Managing Chronic
Kidney Disease

Mary Lauren Ross

© Copyright 2020 - All rights reserved.

The content contained within this book may not be reproduced, duplicated or transmitted without direct written permission from the author or the publisher.

Under no circumstances will any blame or legal responsibility be held against the publisher, or author, for any damages, reparation, or monetary loss due to the information contained within this book, either directly or indirectly.

Legal Notice:

This book is copyright protected. It is only for personal use. You cannot amend, distribute, sell, use, quote or paraphrase any part, or the content within this book, without the consent of the author or publisher.

Disclaimer Notice:

Please note the information contained within this document is for educational and entertainment purposes only. All effort has been executed to present accurate, up to date, reliable, complete information. No warranties of any kind are declared or implied. Readers acknowledge that the author is not engaged in the rendering of legal, financial, medical or professional advice. The content within this book has been derived from various sources. Please consult a licensed professional before attempting any techniques outlined in this book.

By reading this document, the reader agrees that under no circumstances is the author responsible for any losses, direct or indirect, that are incurred as a result of the use of the information contained within this document, including, but not limited to, errors, omissions, or inaccuracies.

TABLE OF CONTENTS

INTRODUCTION 6

CHAPTER 1 7
   HOW DO THE KIDNEYS WORK? 7

CHAPTER 2 15
   CHRONIC KIDNEY DISEASE 15

CHAPTER 3 17
   SLOWING KIDNEY DISEASE 17

CHAPTER 4 20
   ADOPTING A NEW LIFESTYLE TO MINIMIZE YOUR KIDNEY PROBLEMS 20

CHAPTER 5 22
   MANAGING YOUR RENAL DIET WHEN YOU ARE DIABETIC 22

CHAPTER 6 26
   RENAL DIET BASICS 26

CHAPTER 7 30
   HEALTHY AND DELICIOUS RENAL DIET RECIPES BREAKFAST SUGGESTIONS AND IDEAS 30

LUNCH AND PACKED LUNCH IDEAS 33

VEGETARIAN DISHES 39

THE VERSATILE MINCE SECTION 41

CHAPTER 5 42
   RENAL DIET RECIPES 42
      CHICKPEA SALAD 45
      ROQUEFORT PEAR TOAST 46
      SHORTBREAD WITH JAM 47
      SKEWERS OF SEITAN 48
      BEAN SALAD TO SHELL 49
      Raspberry tartlets without gluten 50
      Quiche with ratatouille 51
      Zucchini/shrimp verrines 52
      Homemade sauerkraut 54
      Homemade yogurts with a pressure cooker 55
      Omelet with chicken livers 56
      Cheesecake 57
      Pear and walnut 58
      Potato salad with smoked herring 59
      Salmon with lentils 60

- *Spinach egg cake* 61
- *Cups of strawberries with mango* 62

COCONUT-PINEAPPLE MOUSSE 63

- *Spinach gratin with goat cheese* 64
- *Eggs with milk and goat cheese* 65
- *Palets with squash seeds* 66
- *Whiting bread with sesame* 67
- *Almond/Pear Express Cream* 68
- *Seasonal vegetable cake* 69
- *ZUCCHINI FLAN* 70
- *MUSHROOM CAKE AO-NORI* 71
- *VEGETABLE TOAST* 72
- *Peach fondant* 73
- *Exotic fruit verrines* 74
- *SHORTBREAD WITH JAM* 75
- *Chocolate Pear Charlotte* 76
- *Poached apricots with blackcurrant* 77
- *Bavarian vanilla/coffee* 78
- *CLAFOUTIS MULTI FRUITS* 79
- *LEEK GRATIN* 80
- *GLUTEN-FREE CHOCOLATE FONDANT* 81
- *LIGHT TOMATO PIE* 82
- *OMELET WITH COTTAGE CHEESE AND FRUITS* 83
- *French toast with apples and mint* 84
- *Chicken and Lemon Casserole* 85

SIMPLE MEAT DISHES 86

- *FISH DISHES* 88
- *Kedgeree* 89
- *Tuna Pasta Bake* 90
- *Easy Fish Cakes* 91
- SIDE DISHES 92
  - *Healthy Chips* 92
  - *Dauphinoise Potatoes* 93
  - *PUDDINGS AND CAKES* 94
  - *Syrup Sponge Pudding* 94
  - *Rice Pudding* 95
  - *Apple Crumble* 96
  - *Lemon Cheesecake* 97
  - *Cherry Shortbread* 98
  - *Victoria Sponge Cake* 99
  - *Quick and Easy Flapjacks* 100
  - *Madeira Cake* 101

CHRISTMAS RECIPES 102

- *Brie and Cranberry Filo Parcels* 102
- *Salmon and Chive Paté* 103
- *Sausage and Cranberry Stuffing* 104

 Christmas dinner. *105*
 Jammy Sponge Tarts *106*
 Christmas Cake *107*
 Gingerbread Buche de Noel *108*
 Christmas Pudding *110*

CHAPTER 8 .... **111**
 NUTRITION AND CHRONIC KIDNEY DISEASE 111

CONCLUSION **119**

INTRODUCTION

Chronic renal disease known with the acronym erc is the gradual and permanent loss of functions performed by the kidneys. "It loses its ability to remove waste, to concentrate urine, to maintain the balance of substances in the blood and to maintain a metabolic and hormonal balance that protects every cell in our body.

If the kidneys are damaged, this forces patients to partially replace some of their functions with dialysis or a kidney transplant. The most common causes of this disease are diabetic nephropathy, arterial hypertension and glomerulonephritis. "

This is one of the relevant aspects of the kidney week that will be coordinated by the Chilean nephrology society between May 8 and 14, 2017.

One of the main kidney disease issues is that it can be asymptomatic, being identified only by laboratory tests and kidney scans, and is usually diagnosed using these markers.

Rarely is a renal biopsy necessary and many times it is not possible to determine the disease that caused it. The key signs of renal damage are a rise in creatininemia, uremia and a high protein excretion in the urine.

Renal replacement therapy today has three options: transplantation, peritoneal dialysis, and hemodialysis. Both choices are similar to one another and during his disease a renal patient will go through all of both. The deterioration in the quality of life in those affected generated by this pathology, which can lead them to connect with machines to survive, among other situations of deterioration.

Chronic kidney disease (CKD) is a growing problem worldwide with an estimated incidence of approximately 10 per cent of the population and the majority of early-stage people are unaware of its existence, being able to develop into end-stage kidney disease if there is no intervention.

His prevalence in our country, including all of its phases, is not well documented. In the supposedly healthy adult population, the national health survey measured it at 2.7 percent in 2010. On the other hand, in primary health care consulting patients, the average prevalence of CKD is 12.1%, which is significantly higher in women (14.5%) than in men (7.4).

11 percent are in stage 3; 0.3 percent are in stage 4; and 0.2 percent are in stage 5, which requires dialysis or transplantation. We'll talk about renal diet in this ebook and what you need to know about it.

CHAPTER 1

HOW DO THE KIDNEYS WORK?

Depending on body weight, 4 to 6 litres of blood circulates in the body. Blood is transported to the kidneys through the renal arteries. Every day, about 1,500 litres of blood pass through the kidneys, which are purified by the work of about a million nephrons.

Nephrons consist of small filters called glomeruli that separate water, salts, and impurities from the blood. Protein and blood cells remain in it. The filtered fluid (primary urine) is transported through small channels. There are cells of a particular type (tubular cells) that cause water and salts such as sodium, calcium, phosphorus, and magnesium to return to the blood. The remainder of the fluid is excreted as ultimate urine.

The amount of salt absorbed by the tubular cells depends on blood pressure and the concentration of certain hormones that affect the functioning of these cells. Thus, the kidneys regulate the balance of water and salt in the body. Conversely, the kidneys also have an effect on blood pressure (for example, when blood pressure drops, more water and sodium are secreted into it).

The kidneys also produce a hormone called erythropoietin, which stimulates the production of red blood cells.

What renal failure can cause

Kidney damage can occur either suddenly, and as a result of the long-term disease process. If the kidneys are exposed to the damaging factor for a short time, acute renal failure (ONN) develops, characterized by a rapid increase in creatinine and a decrease in diuresis, and even complete anuria, often requiring renal replacement therapy. This condition can develop in a few hours to 7 days.

Nevertheless, acute failure may result in full recovery within a few months, and it mainly depends on the type of primary disease. However, if the kidney is damaged gradually through the long process of the disease (lasting at least three months) develop chronic kidney disease with the most severe forms: severe chronic kidney failure and end-stage renal disease, requiring dialysis.

Among the factors impairing kidney function are primarily the states of impaired blood flow, specific and non-specific inflammation and immunological factors and substances toxic to the kidneys, all processes can impair urinary tract patency and chronic diseases such as diabetes and hypertension.

Causes of acute renal failure

The factors responsible for acute kidney damage are divided into so-called prerenal, renal, and renal. The first, most common category includes conditions that disturb kidney blood flow, including:

- decreased circulating the blood volume due to haemorrhage, dehydration, excessive diuresis, seepage into the body cavities or extensive burns and injuries;
- heart disease characterized by a sudden decrease in stroke volume;
- states of the sudden increase in the volume of the vascular bed due to a vascular tone disorder (sepsis, antihypertensive, electrolyte disturbances, cirrhosis);

- autoregulation of renal blood flow due to the use of non-steroidal anti-inflammatory drugs, cyclooxygenase inhibitors or angiotensin receptor blockers (drugs used in hypertension);
- conditions of excessive blood viscosity, including hematologic malignancies
- obstruction of the vessels supplying the kidneys due to a blood clot, embolism, aneurysm, external pressure, e.g., by a tumour or inflammation;

Renal factors that damage organ parenchyma include all glomerular inflammatory processes (autoimmune, allergic, viral, bacterial, idiopathic), systemic vasculitis, thrombotic microangiopathy, cholesterol embolism, malignant hypertension, autoimmune diseases including systemic lupus erythematosus and scleroderma systemic, damage to the renal parenchyma due to prolonged impaired blood supply, toxins - including contrast agents and drugs (including ciclosporin, cisplatin, some antibiotics, captopril, methotrexate, indinavir, acyclovir, ethylene glycol and methanol and - attention - popular non-steroidal drugs anti-inflammatory), as well as cancerous infiltrates.

Last but not least, the causes of ONN are conditions that cause obstruction of the urinary tract (also within the bladder) by urolithiasis, blood clots, fragments of damaged nipples, external pressure, e.g. by a cancerous tumour or in diseases of the prostate in men, interruption of the urinary tract or damage to the urethra.

Causes of chronic renal failure

In contrast to ONN, in this disease entity kidney damage occurs gradually, primarily in the course of chronic diseases, such as:

- diabetes mellitus (diabetic nephropathy),
- hypertension (hypertensive nephropathy),
- glomerulonephritis and tubulointerstitial inflammatory processes,
- polycystic degeneration,
- systemic diseases, including sarcoidosis and amyloidosis
- less often long-term impaired blood flow or outflow of urine,
- plasma myeloma,
- HIV nephropathy
- genetically determined syndromes, e.g., Alport syndrome.

The Role of Sodium in the Body

Sodium is one of the elements necessary for the proper functioning of the body. He is primarily responsible for water and electrolyte management, but also has other functions. What are his other roles? Are there serious effects of sodium excess and deficiency? How to introduce a diet that will allow us to reduce sodium intake?

The role of sodium in the body

Sodium has important functions in the body, and disturbances in its concentration can cause serious problems. The main tasks of this valuable element include:

- maintaining the osmotic balance of the body in the extracellular fluids of the body - this means that it regulates the volume of water in the body and protects us from dehydration,
- maintaining acid-base balance (together with potassium and chlorine),

- Involved in the conduction of nerve impulses - sodium is a potassium antagonist, and this element creates a concentration difference on both sides of the cell membrane, thus enabling the transmission of impulses. This process is responsible for the state of smooth muscle, skeletal and heart tension,
- participation in the process of glucose and amino acid transport across cell membranes,
- Activating salivary amylase - a digestive enzyme present in saliva.

Normal sodium concentration in the body is 135-145 mmol /l, and its maintenance is responsible for the renin-angiotensin-aldosterone system. It is a complex hormonal - enzyme system that also regulates the volume of water in the body.

Potassium - role in the body

Potassium belongs to microelements and is an element that performs many essential functions. Thanks to potassium, our cells can transmit electrical impulses, but potassium also helps maintain adequate blood pressure and muscle tone.

Potassium, therefore, is an electrolyte, controls muscle function. It enables the generation of electrical impulses in the cells of our body, including in the cells of the heart muscles, i.e., it is responsible for each heartbeat. Potassium plays the same function in skeletal muscles.

Potassium is a sodium antagonist, and its opposite action consists of, among others, on reducing the volume of extracellular fluids, which helps to control the amount of water in the body. This role of potassium has also associated with the ability to maintain healthy blood pressure by lowering it.

Potassium is involved in the processes in which our cells synthesize proteins, which in turn are muscle building blocks. Thus, potassium is one of the factors that control muscle building and help maintain healthy muscle mass.

Potassium, being also a calcium antagonist, is responsible for proper muscle tone (so-called tonus) by raising their tone.

Also, potassium helps maintain acid-base balance, and thus maintain the homeostasis of the whole body.

Potassium and Our Health

If our body is functioning properly, balance is maintained between potassium and sodium. Disorders in the concentrations of these macroelements cause the occurrence of one of the most common and severe civilization diseases, i.e., hypertension and heart disease. Unlike sodium, low potassium levels promote these diseases.

It is rare that people suffer from potassium deficiency or bearing. This happens, however, in cases where the functioning of our body is disturbed.

Potassium deficiency, or hypokalemia, can occur when we use high blood pressure diuretics, in the case of prolonged vomiting or diarrhoea, and with some kidney problems. Symptoms of hypokalemia are weak, flaccid muscles, arrhythmias, and a slight increase in blood pressure.

Hyperkalemia, which is too high in potassium, causes a dangerous arrhythmia. Hyperkalemia occurs when the kidneys are weak, infections are severe, and when you are taking some heart medicines.

Phosphorus - role in the body

Because as much as 85% of phosphorus is found in bones and teeth, it is necessary to maintain their proper structure. It also occurs in soft tissues and cell membranes, i.e., in the tissues of muscles, heart, and brain. Also plays an essential role in the process of growth and reconstruction or repair of damaged tissues. As one of the elements that take part in the processes occurring in the human body, phosphorus is also an energy transmitter. Thanks to this mineral, food is converted into energy that translates into muscle work.

Phosphorus also ensures the proper functioning of nerves and the brain and is involved in many chemical reactions and metabolic processes in our body. Maintains the overall vitality of the body. In addition, it plays an important role in the work of the heart. For researchers, it is an important carrier of genetic information because it is a component of DNA.

Diet for Kidney Failure : **What to Eat and What to Avoid**

In the diet for renal failure, it is necessary to control the intake of some nutrients such as sodium, phosphorus, potassium, and protein. In the most severe cases where the kidneys are no longer functioning well or in the case of dialysis, it is also necessary to control the number of fluids that are ingested daily. This includes water, juices, and soups.

When talking about kidney failure, it means that the kidneys' ability to filter waste from the blood and form urine is diminished, so it causes specific residues and minerals, such as those mentioned above, to accumulate in the blood and can cause serious consequences, this is due to the restriction of these nutrients in the diet.

So these individuals need to reduce the intake of proteins such as meats, fish, grains, and some types of fruits and legumes such as orange and kiwi. However, in the case of potassium-rich foods, there are some techniques that can be used to reduce the amount of potassium in fruits and vegetables, such as peeling them before eating them.

Foods to be controlled

Renal insufficiency can be acute or chronic, so food restrictions in the diet vary according to the type of inadequacy and the stage in which the disease is found.

Ideally, in these situations, the individual should go to a nutritionist specialized in the area to develop an individual nutritional plan based on the laboratory tests of the person, so the foods mentioned below should be consumed in moderation, since that the fact that they are ingested or not will depend on laboratory values:

1. Foods high in potassium

The kidneys of people with renal insufficiency have difficulty removing excess potassium from the blood, so those people need to control the intake of this mineral by avoiding abuse of them.

Potassium-rich foods are:

- Fruits: avocado, banana, coconut, fig, guava, kiwi, orange, papaya, passion fruit, tangerine, grape, raisins, plums, prune, melon, apricot, blackberries, dates;
- Vegetables: potato, sweet potato, cassava, Creole celery, carrot, chard, beet, celery, cabbage, Brussel sprouts, radish, tomatoes, canned palm, spinach, turnip, and chicory;
- Legumes: beans, lentils, corn, peas, chickpea, soybeans, beans;
- Whole grains: wheat, rice, oats;
- Whole foods: biscuits, whole wheat pasta, breakfast cereals;
- Oleaginous: peanut, cashew, almonds, hazelnuts;
- Industrialized products: chocolate, tomato sauce, meat, and chicken broth tablets;
- Drinks: coconut water, sports drinks, black tea, green tea, matte tea;
- Seeds: sesame, flaxseed;
- Paper or sugar cane guarapo ;
- Salt light

Too much potassium can cause muscle weakness, arrhythmias, and cardiac arrest, so the diet for chronic renal failure has to be individualized and accompanied by

the doctor and the nutritionist, who will evaluate the appropriate amounts of nutrients that each person should ingest.

How to reduce potassium in the food

Some strategies can help reduce the amount of potassium in fruits and vegetables; these are:

- Peel fruits and vegetables;
- Cut and rinse food thoroughly;
- Place the plants to soak in water in the refrigerator for a day, before use;
- Place the food in a pot with water and boil for 10 minutes. Then drain the water and cook again with water and then prepare the food as desired.

Another important suggestion is to avoid the use of pressure cookers and microwaves to prepare meals since these techniques concentrate the potassium content in food by not allowing water to be changed.

2. Foods rich in phosphorus

Phosphorus-rich foods should also be consumed moderately by people with chronic renal failure to control kidney function. These foods are:

- Canned sins;
- Salted, smoked and sausage meats such as sausages and sausages;
- Bacon, bacon;
- Yolk;
- Milk and derivatives;
- Soy and derivatives;
- Beans, lentils, peas, corn;
- Oilseeds such as cashew, almonds, and peanuts;
- Seeds such as sesame and flaxseed;
- Coconut sweet;
- Beer, cola, and hot chocolate.

Symptoms of excess phosphorus are itchy body, hypertension, and mental confusion, and people with kidney failure should keep an eye on these signs.

3. Protein-rich foods

People with chronic renal failure need to control the consumption of proteins because, during their metabolism, toxic wastes are produced that accumulate in the blood, and cannot be eliminated. This is why it is essential to avoid excessive consumption of meat, fish, eggs, milk, and derivatives since they are foods rich in protein.

Ideally, a person with kidney failure should eat one small beef steak at lunch and dinner and one glass of milk or yoghurt per day. However, this amount varies according to how the kidney function is, being more restrictive in those people in whom the kidney almost does not work.

4. Foods rich in salt and water

People with kidney failure also need to control salt intake, since the excess increases blood pressure and forces the kidney to work, further impairing the function of this organ. The same happens with the excess of liquids since these people produce little urine, and the excess of liquids ends up accumulating the organism, causing problems such as swelling and dizziness.

Therefore, the use of:

- Salt;
- Sauces such as ketchup, mayonnaise, aioli, among others;
- Tomato paste;
- Condiments such as cubes, soy sauce, and Worcestershire sauce;
- Canned food and frozen prepared food;
- Snacks, chips, and crackers with salt;
- Fast food;
- Powdered or canned soups.

To avoid excess salt, a good option is to use aromatic herbs to season foods such as parsley, garlic, and basil. The doctor or nutritionist will indicate the appropriate amount of salt and water allowed for each person individually.

How to choose snacks

Restrictions on the feeding of the renal patient can make it difficult to choose snacks. Therefore, the 3 most important recommendations for choosing healthy snacks are:

- Eat always cooked fruit (cook twice), never reusing cooking water, and it must be discarded;
- Restrict industrialized and processed foods that are generally rich in salt or sugars, preferring homemade preparations;
- Avoid the intake of protein foods in snacks.

Diet for acute renal failure

The diet for acute renal failure is usually performed at the hospital level, because it is a situation that occurs suddenly and is treated in the hospital, being carefully calculated by the nutritionist, and may even be necessary to use food through a route intravenously to administer the number of nutrients that the individual requires.

In general, renal function is usually restored, and the individual receives specific instructions on what they can eat to avoid the accumulation of toxins that are eliminated through the kidneys. Normally this diet is usually low in protein, potassium, salt, and phosphorus, as in chronic renal failure, until the function of the kidneys completely returns to normal.

Adapt to renal failure

Discovering that you have kidney failure can be a shock, even if you have known for a long time that your kidneys are not working well. But starting dialysis treatment doesn't have to say that the ones you enjoy are over. It may take a little time to adapt to your new routine, but you are not alone. Your doctors, nurses, and social workers can help you.

Depression and anxiety

Depression is a feeling of sadness that extends for a long time. Anxiety is a feeling of nervousness that comes and goes.

It is normal for you to be nervous when you are going through significant changes in your life, mainly if these changes affect your health and well-being. When you start dialysis treatment, you may have to change your daily routine, your diet, and the type of activities you do. You will probably experience different feelings as you get used to this new lifestyle, such as sadness, fear, regret, and anger. You may not immediately understand what you are feeling, but you may notice that you feel strange.

Symptoms of depression are:
- Changes in sleeping patterns (sleeping too much or having trouble sleeping)
- Loss of interest in those activities you used to enjoy
- Loss of appetite

Some symptoms of anxiety are:
- Heart Rate Acceleration
- Sweating
- breathe too fast
- difficulty thinking about anything except what worries you

You must know that you are not alone. Most people have gone through what you are going through. Many people have felt like you. It is also essential that you know that you do not have to live with these feelings. Help is available. Talk to your social worker about the different ways to start feeling better. You may also find support groups useful.

- **Exercise**

Exercise is a very good way to improve your health. Most people can and should exercise, even if they are undergoing dialysis treatment.

People who exercise regularly feel better, both physically and emotionally. Some benefits of exercise are:
- Mood improvement
- Improvement of heart and lung health
- Weightless
- Joint pain reduction
- Greater flexibility

Exercise does not have to be difficult or painful. In fact, if it hurts to perform a certain exercise, you shouldn't do it! There are many ways to exercise without experiencing pain or discomfort. Consider practising low impact exercises.

These are exercises that do not cause too much tension in the joints. Some examples of low impact exercises are:
- Hike
- Swimming
- Riding a bicycle
- Yoga
- Pilates
- Use of elliptical machine
- Tai Chi
- Stretching
- Climbing stairs

You do not need to join a gym or buy expensive equipment to exercise.

You can walk in your neighbourhood or in the mall. Or you can practice yoga at home on the floor of your living room. Your doctor can help you design an exercise plan that is safe for you, and that suits your dialysis itinerary.

- **Job**

You may be able to continue working during your dialysis treatment. Working can help you feel happier and fulfilled. If you have health insurance through your work, staying in it will help you keep your insurance.

If you want or need to continue working during your dialysis treatment, talk to your doctor about your treatment options. Certain types of dialysis allow you to keep a more flexible schedule during the day.

For example, if you choose night hemodialysis (at night), in the centre or at home, you can perform your dialysis treatments at night, while you sleep. This is also possible with cyclist assisted continuous peritoneal dialysis (CCPD).

If you decide to continue working during your dialysis treatment, it is important that you know your limits. You may feel tired or weak throughout the day. If you receive peritoneal dialysis treatment and make your own exchanges, you must have a clean place in your work to do the exchanges. If you receive hemodialysis treatment, you should not lift heavy objects or put pressure on the arm of your vascular access.

Chapter 2

CHRONIC KIDNEY DISEASE

Chronic kidney disease involves conditions that damage your kidneys and reduce their ability to keep you healthy. If your kidney condition gets worse, waste will build up in your blood to high levels and make you feel sick. Complications such as high blood pressure, weak bones, poor nutritional health, anemia (low blood count), and nerve damage may develop. Also, kidney disease raises the risk of having heart and blood vessel disease. These issues can happen slowly over a long period of time. Diabetes, high blood pressure and other disorders can cause chronic kidney disease. Treatment and early diagnosis will also prevent chronic kidney disease from getting worse. It can ultimately lead to kidney failure as kidney disease progresses, requiring dialysis or a kidney transplant to sustain life.

The Facts About Chronic Kidney Disease (CKD)

- 37 million American adults have Chronic Kidney Disease and millions of others are at increased risk.
- Early detection can help prevent kidney disease from progressing to kidney failure.
- The main cause of death for all persons with CKD is heart disease.
- The best estimate of kidney function is the glomerular filtration rate (GFR).
- Hypertension triggers CKD and hypertension is caused by CKD.
- Persistent proteinuria (protein in urine) indicates CKD is present.
- High-risk categories include those with hypertension, diabetes , and family history of kidney failure.
- There is an increased risk for African Americans , Hispanics, Pacific Islanders, American Indians and seniors.
- CKD can be detected by two basic tests: blood pressure, serum creatinine and urine albumin.

What causes CKD?

Diabetes and high blood pressure are the two primary causes of chronic kidney disease. They are responsible for up to two-thirds of the cases. Diabetes occurs when your blood sugar is too high, causing damage to many of the body's organs, including the kidneys and heart, as well as blood vessels , eyes, and nerves. Hypertension, or high blood pressure, occurs when the pressure of your blood against the walls of your blood vessels increases. High blood pressure may be a leading cause of heart attacks , strokes and chronic kidney disease if uncontrolled, or poorly regulated. Also, chronic kidney disease can lead to high blood pressure.

Other conditions that affect the kidneys are:

- Glomerulonephritis, a group of illnesses that cause the filtering units of the kidney to be inflamed and impaired. These disorders are the third most common kind of kidney disease.
- Inherited diseases, such as polycystic kidney disease, cause the development of large cysts in the kidneys and destroy the tissue surrounding them.
- Malformations that occur when a baby grows in the womb of its mother. For instance, a narrowing may occur that prevents normal urine outflow and causes urine to flow back to the kidney. This causes infections and the kidneys can be damaged.
- Lupus and other diseases that affect the immune system of the body.

- Obstructions caused by disorders in men such as kidney stones, tumors or an enlarged prostate gland.
- Frequent urinary infections.

What are the symptoms of CKD?

Most individuals do not have any significant symptoms until their kidney disease is advanced. However, you may realize that you:

- have trouble concentrating
- feel more tired and have less energy
- have muscle cramping at night
- have a poor appetite
- have swollen feet and ankles
- have trouble sleeping
- have puffiness around your eyes, especially in the morning
- need to urinate more often, especially at night.
- have dry, itchy skin

Anyone can get chronic kidney disease at any age. Some individuals are, however, more likely to develop kidney disease than others. You could be at increased risk of developing kidney disease if you:

- have high blood pressure
- have diabetes
- are older
- have a family history of kidney failure
- belong to a population group that has high blood pressure or high rate of diabetes, such as Hispanic Americans, African Americans, Asian, American Indians, and Pacific Islanders.

Chapter 3

SLOWING KIDNEY DISEASE

Having your kidneys function — even a little — can help you feel better and live longer. You will delay the need for treatment for kidney failure if you can slow your CKD. The kinds of improvements you might make to improve your heart, or your kidneys will also be helped by the rest of your body. Here are several things that you should do or avoid to protect your kidneys:

Blood sugar meter

Maintain the blood sugar within the target range. Blood vessels, including nephrons in the kidneys, are affected by high blood sugar. Your doctor will give you a target for fasting blood sugar if you have diabetes and for two hours after you eat. Test your blood sugar regularly to see how it changes depending on what you eat and how active you are. If you haven't done this yet, cut down on added sugar and processed carbs, such as bread, cakes, and rice. Take walks or find other ways to be active. Take your diabetes medicine(s) as prescribed.

- Maintain your blood pressure in the target range given to you by your doctor, too. Even if your blood pressure has been low throughout your life, it may now be high and it may be difficult to regulate. In CKD, it is common to require more than one drug for blood pressure. Check your blood pressure at home. Keep a log of the results so that you can tell your care team when it is high or low and what time you take your blood pressure pills. If you have side effects, speak with your doctor; a different medicine could work better for you. Exercise can also help reduce blood pressure.
- Lose Weight If You Are Overweight. The ten-year CARDIA study of young individuals (average age of 35) discovered that the more people weighed, the faster their kidney function decreased. This was true even though they did not have high blood pressure or diabetes. It's hard to lose weight, but it can be done, and it can work in a lot of ways. Ask for your care team's assistance if you need it.
- Don't drink soda. Drinking one or more sodas daily has been linked to kidney damage according to a large study. A second study discovered that two or more diet sodas a day can lead to kidney damage or make it progress faster.
- If you smoke or use street drugs, try to stop! Kidneys may be affected by smoking and most street drugs. If quitting was easy, of course, everybody would do it. There are a variety of ways to stop smoking, from going cold turkey to patches, e-cigarettes, or nicotine gum. Even cutting back may help. You may need a rehab program if you use street drugs. Talk to your care team if you need help to stop a habit that is affecting your health.
- Balance your blood pH. A healthy blood pH is between 7.38 and 7.42. When the kidneys don't function well, they will fail to maintain the acid-base balance in your body. Acid can build up from protein foods you eat. Grains and protein foods such as eggs, dairy, meat, beans, and peas form acid wastes then they break down. Your body requires protein for muscles and self–repair. Most of us, though, consume a lot more protein than we need. One way to make the kidneys last

longer, at least if you are older, is to have a low-acid diet (with lots of veggies). Ask your doctor if you can help protect your kidneys with sodium bicarbonate, too.

Examples of dairy products

- Eat Less Protein. This forms blood urea nitrogen (BUN) as protein breaks down. It is difficult on the kidneys to extract BUN. You produce less BUN when you consume less protein, which can help your kidneys last a little longer. Research has shown that it may benefit much more to consume very little protein, but this is difficult to do and there is a risk of malnutrition.
- Eat Less Phosphorus. Phosphorus is present in meat, dairy, nuts, poultry, fish, beans, and cola drinks. Weak kidneys are unable to get as much phosphorus out of your blood. When your levels are too high, it can make your bones fragile.
- Limit Shellfish. Studies have shown that in mice, a toxin called domoic acid in shellfish and certain fish eating algae can damage the kidneys. People aren't mice. But, the really alarming result was that the kidneys could be affected by very small amounts of the toxin. Shellfish also have high purine levels, which, if you have gout, can be a concern. So, if you eat a lot, it might be prudent to cut back on shellfish.
- Skip Canned Foods. In the United States, most food cans are filled with bisphenol A (BPA). BPA has been associated with high blood pressure, diabetes, and obesity. Most packaged foods tend to have a very high salt or sugar content and are often highly processed. Glass jars or shelf safe cartons do not have BPA.
- Avoid Certain Pain Pills." Non–steroidal anti–inflammatory drugs" (NSAIDs) like Aleve®, Motrin®, and Advil® can cause kidney damage. Kidneys need a strong blood flow to function. NSAIDs minimize the flow of blood into and out of the kidneys. It takes years of everyday use for NSAIDs to cause CKD, in most cases. But NSAIDs will make it get worse faster, once CKD is present. Speak to your doctor about pain relief options that won't hurt your kidneys any further. If you take one tablet here and there and your kidneys are still functioning, drink a full glass of water with it.
- Need A Contrast Dye X – ray? Ask For Kidney Precautions. Dye that is injected into a vein for a CT or MRI scan will pass through your kidneys. Kidney damage may be caused by a dye called gadolinium. This dye can also cause an unusual problem called nephrogenic systemic fibrosis. NSF can be fatal, and can make the skin and organs thicken. There is no treatment for NSF. If a doctor orders an X-ray dye examination, ask if there are other ways to discover the same things. Would an ultrasound work, instead? Be sure to tell the radiologist about your CKD if you need to have a comparison. He or she might be able to dilute the dye or to wash it out of your blood by giving you an IV with sodium bicarbonate.
- Antioxidants May Help You. Every cell in the human body needs oxygen. But, excess oxygen in the wrong places can "oxidize" and cause damage, much like rust. Antioxidants may help your kidneys and it help protect your cells. Ask your doctor if antioxidants might be worth taking:
    - Turmeric
    - Coenzyme Q10

CKD is a risk factor for stroke and heart disease. The heart and blood vessels often appear to be affected by the same diseases that affect the kidneys. The good news is that moving gets your blood flowing, which boosts your kidneys' blood flow, and helps your heart. So, exercise is a win-win for your body. It can also help to slow the CKD rate.

The goal is thirty minutes of active movement daily. And, the thirty minutes don't have to be all at once. You can split your exercise into ten-minute blocks if you like.

Thinking of starting an exercise plan? If it is been a while since you were active, first speak with your doctor. Start slow, and build up distance, time, or weight slowly. Track your progress in order to see how you are doing. You can even set targets and reward yourself when you reach them.

Exercise doesn't have to be on a machine at a pricey gym. Here are some other alternatives you may think about, and you can come up with more:

- Walking is great exercise, and if you have a loved one as a companion, you get time together. You can enjoy an outdoor stroll if the weather is good and you live in a safe place. Or, a lot of people walk in malls or at indoor tracks so they do not miss out. A jog-walk will give you a more vigorous workout (trading off walking and jogging).
- Take Up a Sport. From tennis to badminton to bowling, you can spend time with others and improve your fitness at the same time if there's a team sport you like.
- Do a little work. Paint a wall or a fence. Get out and pull any weeds or cut the shrubs in the yard. Use a push mower to mow the grass. Vacuum a couple of rooms. You will get something done, be active, and feel good about yourself.
- Dance, Skate, Play! Moving is moving, whether you jump on a trampoline, paddle a canoe or take your partner out for a spin. Think of what you liked as a kid-it might give you some ideas of things to try.

Chapter 4

ADOPTING A NEW LIFESTYLE TO MINIMIZE YOUR KIDNEY PROBLEMS

Kidney diseases are silent killers that can affect the quality of life to a large extent. There are many ways that the risk of developing kidney disease can be reduced.

Keep fit, Be active

This will help maintain the optimum weight of your body, decrease your blood pressure, and reduce your risk of Chronic Kidney Disease.

The idea of "On the move for kidney health" is a joint march around the world involving the public, celebrities and practitioners walking, running and cycling around a public field. Why not join them!

Eat a healthy diet

This will help maintain an optimum weight for the body, minimize blood pressure, heart disease, prevent diabetes, and other Chronic Kidney Disease-related conditions.

Reduce your salt consumption. 5-6 grams of salt per day is the optimal sodium intake. This includes the salt already in your foods. Try to minimize the amount of processed and restaurant food and do not add salt to food in order to reduce the salt intake. Controlling your salt consumption would be easier if you cook the food yourself with fresh ingredients.

Check and control your blood sugar

About half of people with diabetes are unaware that they have diabetes. As part of your general body checkup, you therefore need to check your blood sugar level. For those who are approaching middle age or older, this is particularly important. Around half of people with diabetes experience kidney damage, but if the diabetes is well managed, this can be prevented / limited. Check your kidney function regularly with urine and blood tests.

Check and control your blood pressure

About half of people with high blood pressure are unaware that they have high blood pressure. As part of your general body checkup, you therefore need to check your blood pressure. For those who are reaching middle age or older, this is particularly important. Your kidneys can be impaired by high blood pressure. This is particularly probable in conjunction with other causes, such as diabetes , cardio-vascular diseases and high cholesterol. With good blood pressure control, the risk can be decreased.

The level of normal adult blood pressure is 120/80. Hypertension is diagnosed if the systolic blood pressure readings on both days reach ~140 mmHg and/or the diastolic blood pressure readings on both days reach ~90 mmHg (WHO) when measured on two different days.

If your blood pressure is persistently above the average range (especially if you are a young person), you should contact your doctor to address the risks, the need for lifestyle change and medication treatment.

The recommendations for high blood pressure (2017) were updated by the American Heart Association and the American College of Cardiology and indicated that high blood pressure should be treated sooner with lifestyle modifications and treatment at 130/80 mm Hg instead of 140/90 mm Hg. This suggestion, however, has not been accepted by all health organizations around the world. It's best to see a doctor.

Take appropriate fluid intake

For any individual, the right amount of fluid intake depends on several variables, including health conditions, pregnancy, breastfeeding, exercise, and climate.

In a comfortable climate, this typically means 8 cups, around 2 liters (quarts) per day for a healthy person.

This needs to be changed when the climate condition is severe. If you have kidney disease or liver or heart disease, you may need to alter your fluid intake. Consult your doctor about the fluid intake that is appropriate for your condition.

Don't smoke

Smoking slows down the flow of blood to the kidneys. It may decrease their ability to function normally as less blood enters the kidneys. Smoking also raises the risk of kidney cancer by about 50%.

Do not take over-the-counter pain-killer/anti-inflammatory tablets regularly.

Common drugs such as non-steroidal anti-inflammatory (NSAIDS)/ pain killers (for instance, drugs such as ibuprofen) can damage the kidneys if taken frequently.

Taking only a couple of doses will damage your kidneys if you have kidney disease or reduced kidney function. Consult your doctor or pharmacist if in doubt.

Get your kidney function checked, If you have one or more of the 'high risk' factors.

- you have hypertension
- you have diabetes
- you have a family history of kidney disease
- you are obese

Chapter 5

MANAGING YOUR RENAL DIET WHEN YOU ARE DIABETIC

One of the most effective therapies in the managing kidney disease and diabetes is diet. You will need to work with a dietitian to develop an eating plan that's right for you if you have been diagnosed with kidney disease as a result of diabetes. This strategy will help control the levels of blood glucose and reduce the amount of waste and fluid processed by the kidneys.

Which nutrients do I need to regulate?

Your dietician will provide you with dietary instructions that tell you how much protein, fat , and carbohydrates you will consume, and how much potassium, sodium, and phosphorus you can consume each day. Since these minerals need to be lower in your diet, you can restrict or eliminate those foods when planning your meals.

Portion control is also important. Speak with your dietitian about tips for measuring a serving size accurately. What can be measured on a regular diet as one serving may count as three servings on the kidney diet.

In order to maintain your blood glucose at an even level, the doctor and dietitian will also recommend that you eat meals and snacks of the same size and carbohydrate/calorie content at certain times of the day. It is vital that blood glucose levels are always tested and the results are shared with your doctor.

What can I eat?

An example of food choices that are commonly recommended on a standard renal diabetic diet is given below. This list is focused on the inclusion of foods containing sodium , phosphorus, potassium, and high sugar content. Ask your dietitian if you can have any of the listed foods and ensure you know what the recommended serving size should be.

Carbohydrate Foods

Milk and nondairy

RECOMMENDED	AVOID
Non-dairy creamer, plain yogurt, skim or fat-free milk, sugar-free pudding, sugar-free ice cream, sugar-free yogurt, sugar-free nondairy frozen desserts* *Portions of dairy products are often limited to four ounces due to high potassium, phosphorus or protein content	Buttermilk, sweetened yogurt, chocolate milk, sugar sweetened, sugar sweetened ice cream, pudding, sugar sweetened nondairy frozen desserts

Breads and starches

RECOMMENDED	AVOID
Sourdough, whole grain bread and whole wheat, unsweetened, white, wheat, rye, cream of wheat, grits, malt-o-meal, rice, bagel (small), refined dry cereals, noodles, white or whole wheat pasta, cornbread (made from scratch), flour tortilla, hamburger bun, unsalted crackers	Frosted or sugar-coated cereals, bran bread, gingerbread, pancake mix, cornbread mix, instant cereals, bran or granola, biscuits, salted snacks including: potato chips, corn chips and crackers Whole wheat cereals like oatmeal, wheat flakes and raisin bran, and whole grain hot cereals contain more potassium and phosphorus than refined products.

Fruits and juices

RECOMMENDED	AVOID
Applesauce, apricot halves, apples, apple juice, berries including: cranberries, blackberries and blueberries, strawberries, raspberries, low sugar cranberry juice, grapes, grape juice, kumquats, cherries, fruit cocktail, grapefruit, plums, tangerine, watermelon, mandarin oranges, pears, pineapple, fruit canned in unsweetened juice	Bananas, cantaloupe, avocados, dried fruits including: raisins, dates, and prunes, kumquats, star fruit, fresh pears, honeydew melon, kiwis, mangos, oranges and orange juice, papaya, nectarines, pomegranate, fruit canned in syrup

Starchy vegetables

RECOMMENDED	AVOID
Mixed vegetables with corn and peas (eat these less often because they are high in phosphorus), corn, peas, potatoes (soaked to reduce potassium)	Yams, baked beans, baked potatoes, sweet potatoes, dried beans (kidneys, pinto or soy, lima, lentil), succotash, winter squash, pumpkin

Non-starchy vegetables

RECOMMENDED	AVOID
Brussels sprouts, carrots, asparagus, beets, broccoli, cabbage, cauliflower, celery, cucumber, green beans, iceberg lettuce, eggplant, frozen broccoli cuts, kale, leeks, red and green peppers, mustard	Beet greens, cactus, cooked Chinese cabbage, Artichoke, fresh bamboo shoots, kohlrabi, rutabagas, tomatoes, tomato

greens, okra, onions, radishes, raw spinach (1/2 cup), summer squash, turnips, snow peas	sauce or paste, sauerkraut, cooked spinach, tomato juice, vegetable juice

Higher-protein foods

Meats, cheeses and eggs

RECOMMENDED	AVOID
Lean cuts of meat, fish, poultry, and seafood; eggs, low cholesterol egg substitute; cottage cheese (limited due to high sodium content)	Bacon, cheeses, hot dogs, canned and luncheon meats, organ meats, salami, salmon, sausage, nuts, pepperoni

Higher-fat foods

Seasoning and calories

RECOMMENDED	AVOID
Tub or soft margarine low in trans fats, cream cheese, low fat mayonnaise, mayonnaise, sour cream, low fat cream cheese, low fat sour cream	Bacon fat, Crisco®, lard, shortening, back fat, butter, margarines high in trans fats, whipping cream

Beverages

RECOMMENDED	AVOID
Water, diet clear sodas, lemonade sweetened or homemade tea with an artificial sweetener	Regular or diet dark colas, fruit-flavored drinks or water sweetened with fruit juices, beer, fruit juices, bottled or lemonade containing sugar or or canned iced tea, syrup, or phosphoric acid; tea or lemonade sweetened with real sugar

You may also be instructed to avoid or limit the following salty and sweet foods:

- Honey

- Molasses
- Baked goods
- Candy
- Canned foods
- Condiments
- Onion, garlic or table salt
- Chocolate Regular sugar
- Syrup
- Ice cream
- TV dinners
- Meat tenderizer
- Salted chips and snacks
- Marinades
- Nuts
- Pizza

Chapter 6

RENAL DIET BASICS

Eating correctly is important for kidney health. Those with kidney disease need to monitor the consumption of potassium, sodium, and phosphorus especially.

People with kidney disease may also need to control some important nutrients. The following information will help you modify your diet. Please discuss your individual and specific diet needs with your dietitian or doctor.

Some substances that are crucial for monitor or promote a renal diet are listed below:

Sodium

Sodium is a mineral (sodium chloride) present in salt and is commonly used in food preparation. Salt is one of the seasonings that is most frequently used, and it takes time to get used to reducing the salt in your diet. Salt / sodium reduction, however, is an effective aid in controlling the kidney disease.

The role of sodium in the body?

Sodium is a mineral found in most natural foods. The majority of individuals think of salt and sodium as interchangeable. Salt, however, is a compound of sodium and chloride. The food we eat may contain salt, or may contain other types of sodium. Processed foods contain higher levels of sodium due to added salt.

Sodium is one of the three main electrolytes in the body (the other two being potassium and chloride). The fluids going into and out of the tissues and cells of the body are regulated by electrolytes. Sodium contributes to:

- Regulating blood volume and blood pressure
- Regulating muscle contraction and nerve function
- Balancing how much fluid the body eliminates or keeps
- Regulating the acid-base balance of blood

Why should sodium intake be monitored by kidney patients? For people with kidney disease, too much sodium can be dangerous because their kidneys can not remove excess sodium and fluid from the body adequately. As sodium and fluid build up in the tissues and bloodstream, they may cause:

- High blood pressure
- Increased thirst
- Edema: swelling in the face, hands, and legs
- Shortness of breath: fluid can build up in the lungs, making it very difficult to breathe
- Heart failure: excess fluid in the bloodstream can overwork your heart, making it weak and enlarged

How can patients monitor their sodium intake?

- Make sure you read food labels. Sodium content is always listed. Avoid foods containing more than 300 mg of sodium per serving (or 600 mg for a full frozen meal). Avoid foods that have salt in the first four or five items in the ingredient list.

- Use fresh, instead than packaged meats.
- Pay close attention to serving sizes.
- Avoid processed foods.
- Choose fresh vegetables and fruits or no-salt-added frozen and canned produce.
- Use spices that do not list "salt" in their title (choose garlic powder instead of garlic salt.)
- Compare brands and use items that are lowest in sodium.
- Limit total sodium content to 400 mg per meal and 150 mg per snack.
- Don't use salt when cooking food.
- Don't put salt on food when you eat.
- Do not eat ham, hot dogs, bacon, sausage, lunch meet, chicken tenders or nuggets, or regular canned soup. Eat only soups that have labels indicating a decrease in the sodium level, and eat only one cup-not the entire can.
- Canned vegetables should indicate "no salt added".
- Don't use flavored salts such as onion salt, garlic salt, or "seasoned" salt. Also, avoid sea salt or koshe.
- Make sure you look for lower salt or "no salt added" options for your favorite foods such as box mixes or peanut butter.
- Don't purchase frozen or refrigerated meats that are packaged "in a solution"; or pre-seasoned. These items are usually pork chops, pork tenderloin, chicken breasts, burgers, or steaks.

Potassium

Potassium is a mineral that is involved in how muscles function. Potassium builds up in the blood when the kidneys don't function properly. This can cause changes, perhaps even leading to a heart attack, in how the heart beats. Potassium is primarily present in vegetables and fruits, plus meat and milk. You will need to avoid some of them and limit the number of others.

Potassium-rich foods to avoid:

- Melons such as honeydew and cantaloupe (watermelon is okay)
- Grapefruit juice
- Prune juice
- Bananas
- Oranges and orange juice
- Tomatoes, tomato sauce, tomato juice
- Pumpkin
- Winter squash
- Dried beans – all kinds
- Cooked greens, collards, Swiss Chard, spinach, kale

Other foods to avoid include granola, molasses, bran cereals, "salt substitute" or "lite" salt. To encourage you to eat them in SMALL quantities, potatoes and sweet potatoes need special handling. Peel them, cut them into small slices or cubes, and soak them in a large amount of water for several hours. Pour off the soaking water when you are about to cook them and use a good amount of water in the pan. Before you prepare them to feed, drain the water. To avoid getting too much potassium, make sure to eat a large variety of fruits and vegetables every day. What is potassium in the body and its role? Potassium is a mineral present in many of the foods that we consume and is naturally found in the body as well. Potassium plays a vital role I n keeping the heartbeat normal and the muscles functioning correctly. Potassium is also necessary for the maintenance of fluid and electrolyte balance in the bloodstream, . The kidneys help to keep the body's proper amount of potassium and remove unnecessary amounts into the urine.

Why should kidney patients monitor their potassium consumption?

When the kidneys fail, they can no longer extract excess potassium, so potassium levels build up in the body. High blood potassium is known as hyperkalemia, which can trigger:

- An irregular heart beat
- Slow pulse
- Heart attacks
- Muscle weakness
- Death

How can patients monitor their potassium consumption?

A patient must control the amount of potassium that reaches the body when the kidneys no longer regulate potassium.

Tips to help keep potassium levels in your blood safe, make sure you:

- Speak with a renal dietitian about developing an eating plan.
- Reduce the consumption of foods that are high in potassium.
- Limit dairy and milk products to 8 oz per day.
- Choose fresh vegetables and fruits.
- Avoid salt substitutes and seasonings with potassium.
- Read labels on packaged foods and avoid potassium chloride.
- Keep a food journal.
- Pay attention to serving size.

Phosphorus

Phosphorus is another mineral that will build up in your blood when your kidneys don't function properly. Calcium can be extracted from your bones when this occurs and can settle in your skin or blood vessels. Bone disease may then become an issue, making you more likely to get a break in the bone.

- Dairy foods are the main source of phosphorus in the diet, so limit milk to one cup daily. If you use cheese or yogurt instead of liquid milk – only one container OR one ounce a day!
- Some vegetables contain phosphorus too. Limit these to one cup per WEEK: greens, broccoli, dried beans, Brussels sprouts, and mushrooms.
- Certain cereals need to be limited to one serving a week: wheat cereals, bran, granola, and oatmeal.
- White bread is better than crackers or whole grain breads.
- Phosphorus is also present in soft drinks, so only drink clear ones. Don't drink Mountain Dew® (any kind), root beers, colas, Dr. Pepper® (any kind). Avoid Hawaiian Punch®, Cool® iced tea, Fruitworks®, and Aquafina® tangerine pineapple.
- Avoid all kinds of beers, because they contain phosphorus.

What is Phosphorus and its role in the body?

Phosphorus is a mineral essential in the maintenance and growth of bones. Phosphorus also helps grow connective tissue and organs and assists in the movement of muscles. When phosphorus-containing food is eaten and digested, phosphorus is removed by the small intestines so that it can be stored in the bones.

Why should kidney patients monitor Phosphorus consumption?

Normal functioning kidneys can remove extra phosphorus in your blood. The kidneys no longer expel excess phosphorus when kidney function is compromised. High levels of phosphorus can pull calcium from your bones, making them weak. This also results in toxic deposits of calcium in the blood vessels, eyes, lungs, and heart.

How can patients monitor their Phosphorus consumption?

Phosphorus can be present in many foods. Therefore, patients with impaired kidney function should function with a renal dietitian to help manage phosphorus levels.

Tips to help maintain phosphorus at safe levels:

- Know what foods are low in phosphorus.
- Pay careful attention to servings size
- Eat smaller amounts of food that are rich in protein at meals and for snacks.
- Eat fresh vegetables and fruits.
- Ask your doctor about using phosphate binders at meal time.
- Avoid packaged foods that contain added phosphorus. Look for the words with "PHOS" on ingredient labels.
- Keep a food journal

Protein

Protein isn't a problem for healthy kidneys. Normally, protein is consumed and waste products are created, which in turn are filtered by the nephrons of the kidney. Then, the waste turns into urine with the aid of additional renal proteins. Damaged kidneys, on the other hand, fail to eliminate protein waste and it accumulates in the blood. For Chronic Kidney Disease patients, proper protein intake is tricky as the amount varies with each stage of the disease. Protein is necessary for the preservation of tissues and other bodily roles, so it is vital to consume the prescribed amount for the particular stage of disease according to your renal dietician or nephrologist.

Fluids

Fluid control is essential for patients in the later stages of Chronic Kidney Disease because normal fluid intake can lead to fluid build-up in the body that could become harmful. People on dialysis also have reduced production of urine, so increased fluid in the body can place undue pressure on the heart and lungs of the person. A patient's fluid allowance is measured on an individual basis, based on urine production and dialysis settings. It is essential to follow your nephrologist's/nutritionist's fluid consumption guidelines. To regulate the intake of fluids, patients should:

- Not drink more than what your doctor orders
- Be aware of the amount of fluids used in cooking
- Count all foods that will melt at room temperature

Chapter 7

HEALTHY AND DELICIOUS RENAL DIET RECIPES BREAKFAST SUGGESTIONS AND IDEAS

Welcome to the breakfast segment. This section is intended to give you some ideas if you are bored or stuck with breakfast cereals and toast.

Fruit Salad and Yoghurt

This recipe uses tinned fruit instead of fresh, which is excellent if you are on a potassium limit as tinned fruit is naturally lower in potassium-just remember to skim the juice off as this is where much of the potassium is.

Serves one

- Tinned fruit, such as pears, peaches or perhaps a fruit cocktail. Pick the ones tinned in juice if you need to lose weight or you are diabetic, otherwise you can try the ones in syrup.
- Yogurt of your choice. Go for low-fat or fat-free yogurt if you're trying to lose weight. On the other hand, choose the full fat / thick and creamy yoghurt if you are struggling to keep your weight up.

Note- you would need to count the yogurt as part of your 1/2 pint (300ml) milk allowance if you are on a phosphate restriction (for example, a 125 g yogurt is equivalent to 125ml of milk).

The Bread Basket

Most plain breads are low in potassium and phosphate, so here are some recommendations on the variety of plain breads available for breakfast. Opt for wholemeal varieties where possible. These breads can be served with: cream cheese (which is low in phosphate), butter, honey, syrup, jam, marmalade or an egg cooked to your liking.

- Brioche*
- Ready-made shop bought breakfast pancakes
- Crumpets (low in phosphates so have only occasionally)
- English muffin
- Plain bagel
- Butter croissants*

* These products are higher in fat, so if you are trying to lose weight, be careful.

Traditional Cooked English Breakfast

Due to the high phosphate and potassium products it contains, many people avoid a typical cooked breakfast, but a cooked breakfast can still be enjoyed occasionally by complying with these guidelines.

Serves one

- One egg – any way you like
- Two pieces of bacon or one sausage (opt for low fat or remove fat if trying to lose weight)
- Four small mushrooms or one small tomato or two tbsp of baked beans
- As much toast as you like (however, be careful if you want to lose weight)

Preparation method

1. Grilling is the ideal cooking method if you are trying to lose weight, or you can fry with minimal oil in a non-stick frying pan or use spray oil.
2. Frying in fat will help increase the calories of your breakfast If you need to gain weight then.

High Energy Porridge

If you are underweight or accidentally lose weight, this high energy recipe is useful because it contains loads of extra calories.

Remember – if you are on a phosphate or fluid restriction then the milk should be excluded from your daily allowance for milk and fluid.

Serves One

- 35g (1¼oz) porridge oats
- 200ml full fat milk
- Optional: add cream and syrup or jam for extra energy

Preparation method

1. Mix all ingredients in a pan, heat the pan and boil for three to four minute.

2. Alternatively cook in the microwave for around one to two minutes, stirring at thirty second intervals.

Healthy Porridge

This porridge can be a healthy choice if you are ready to lose weight, since it is low in calories and high in fiber, which will make you stay full for longer, so you are less likely to snack before lunch. You may want to try rice or soya milk to supplement the skimmed milk if you are on a phosphate restriction since it is naturally lower in phosphate as well as low in fat.

Serves 1

- 100ml skimmed milk
- 35g (1¼oz) porridge oats
- Sprinkle of cinnamon
- ½ grated apple
- 100ml water

Preparation method

1. Mix all ingredients in a pan, heat the pan and boil for three to four minutes.

2. Alternatively cook in the microwave for around one to two minutes, stirring at

thirty second intervals.

Homemade Granola

Many shop bought granolas are unsuited if you are following phosphate and potassium restrictions due to the high content of dried fruit and nuts. To make your own alternative oat meal, here is an simple recipe that can be served with yogurt, stewed fruits, or milk. Here we have added dried cranberries as they are lower in potassium than other dried fruits; however, it will taste equally good without.

Makes up to ten servings

- Four tablespoons of vegetable oil or sunflower oil
- One lemon juice table spoon
- Two tablespoons of brown soft sugar
- Two tablespoons clear honey or golden syrup
- Dried cranberries (optional)
- 300g (10½oz) rolled oats

Preparation method

1. Preheat the oven to 140 ° C (120 ° C Fan)/275 ° F / Gas 1.
2. The oil, syrup/honey, lemon juice and sugar are melted in a large saucepan over a low heat. The intention is not to allow the mixture to bubble, only to allow the ingredients to melt and blend together. Then add the oats and stir thoroughly.
3. Spread the mixture in an even layer on a baking tray (depending on their size, you will need two baking trays. Bake in the oven until crisp for around 30-40 minutes. Check the granola every ten minutes and stir to ensure an even bake.
4. You can add a few handfuls of dried cranberries once cooked and cooled. The granola should be kept in an airtight container and utilized within one month.

LUNCH AND PACKED LUNCH IDEAS

Going out and about while on a dietary restriction doesn't have to be challenging. This lunch section provides kidney friendly suggestions that you can have both at home and away.

Pasta, Rice, or Couscous Salad

Pasta, rice, and couscous are low potassium alternatives to potato and make a filling alternative to bread.

Try cold cooked rice, couscous, or pasta mixed with ham, chicken, or tuna, and a range of

vegetables such as olives, peppers, sweet corn, cucumber, and some mayo. You could try flavoring it with some spices or herbs, for instancepaprika, curry powder, dried basil, or parsley. A dash of salad dressing, stirring in soft white cream cheese or spoonful of pesto can give it that extra flavor.

Oatcake or Rice Cake Toppings

Rice cakes and Oat can be used as a healthy snack. Below are some suggestions for healthy toppings, which are also low in phosphate and potassium.

- Cottage cheese mixed with peas (canned or pre-boiled), tuna, and thyme
- Cottage cheese mixed with sweet corn (canned), or mixed with pineapple (drained and canned)
- Lean ham topped with cream cheese
- Cream cheese mixed with chive and garlic or parsley, or any other spice or herb
- Tinned fish (without the bones as this makes them high in phosphate)
- Egg mayonnaise
- Tuna mayonnaise

Sandwiches

Sandwiches could consist of wraps, rolls, bread, pitta, or any other variety of bread available these days. The better alternative is always wholemeal because it contains more fibre. However, if you prefer white then go for this occasionally. Here are some recommended fillings that provide great sources of protein perfect for dialysis patients:

- Cream and Ham cheese
- Mayonnaise and Chicken pesto
- Coronation chicken (chicken mixed with mayonnaise and some curry powder)
- Tuna mayo with cucumber
- Cheese (within allowance), a small amount of mayonnaise and salad
- Cress and Egg
- Horseradish,sliced beef or mustard
- Cranberry and Brie
- Cheese (within allowance) and coleslaw

- Chutney, lettuce, and vegetarian sausage
- Sliced falafel with chilli sauce, shredded lettuce, and spring onions
- Mozzarella, basil, roasted red peppers, and garlic mayonnaise
- Cucumber and cream cheese
- Cranberry sauce and turkey with lettuce

Quiche

Since quiche is made from eggs that are a good source of protein, quiche is a good lunch to replace the protein lost during dialysis.

Ready-made quiches are fine, but opt for low / reduced salt alternatives (less than 1.5 g per 100g). If you want to lose weight, then you might want to skip the pastry and prepare your own quiche utilizing the 'pastry-less quiche recipe' in the vegetarian section of this book.

Other Lunch Box Snacks

- Fruit such as orange, apple, pear (best option if you're trying to lose weight)
- Yogurt (within milk allowance if you are on a restriction) (try fat free or low fat varieties if you are trying to lose weight)
- Corn crisp e.g. Monster Munch, Quavers, Skips, Dorritos, Wotsits, poppadoms, Tortilla chips (if you are trying to lose weight choose low calorie alternatives e.g. around 100kcal per packet).
- Crisps are high in salt, therefore limit the number of times you enjoy these.
- Mini packets of breadsticks
- Butter or plain popcorn (avoid the butter variety if you are trying to lose weight)
- Mini rice cakes, snackajacks, plain crackers e.g. water biscuits
- Plain biscuits eg Short bread, Rich Tea, or Digestives
- Cereal bar (avoid any containing dried fruit or nuts)
- Flap jacks (can be high in fat if you are trying to lose weight)
- Prawn crackers
- Muffins

What about Chocolate?

Chocolate is very high in phosphate and potassium regardless of whether it is milk, dark or white chocolate, so if you're on a phosphate and/or potassium restriction, it's best to eat in moderation. If you choose to have some chocolate as an occasional treat, then opting for something that contains small amount of chocolate is preferable than eating chunks of chocolate. For instance, the following foods all contain chocolate in small quantities:

- Chocolate digestives biscuits.

- Small chocolate bar (wafer or biscuit based such as a Kitkat, Penguin, or Taxi as they have less of the high phosphate chocolate).

- Chocolate chip cookie (avoid double choc chip)

- Chocolate chip muffin or cake (not double choc chip)

- Chocolate chip cereal bar

Soups, Snacks, and Starters

Goat's Cheese Rarebit

Do not be put off by the use of goat's cheese and soya milkin this recipe – they're both much lower in phosphate than cheddar and cow's milks and are equally tasty.

Serves two-four

- 25g (¾oz) flour
- 25g (¾oz) olive oil, butter or vegetable spread
- 175g (6oz) soft goat's cheese
- Four slices bread
- 150ml soya milk (we used unsweetened)
- Two egg yolks
- ½ tsp mustard
- Pepper

Preparation method

1. Place the butter or spread, cheese and soya milkin a saucepan and heat until melted and smooth.
2. Stir in the flour, then bring the mixture to a boil, stir continuously while it thickens, .
3. Remove from the heat and add the pepper and mustard. Leave for five minutes to cool, then mix in the egg yolks with a fork.
4. Toast the bread on one side, turn over and split the rarebit blend between the slices.
5. Put under a hot grill and cook until golden and bubbling.

Pesto Cream Veggie Dip

This dip recipe is perfect as a small meal, a dip to share with friends, or as a snack. Using cream cheese makes it low in phosphate and if served with crackers, corn crisps, or toasted pitta bread,instead than potato crisps they would be low in potassium too.

- 100g (3½oz) cream cheese
- 200g (7oz) basil pesto
- Two tablespoons parmesan cheese
- 100g (3½oz) sour cream

Preparation method

1. Place cream cheese, sour cream, pesto and parmesan cheese in a bowl and stir well.
2. Stir until chill and creamy. Ready to serve.

Smoked Mackerel Paté

Enjoy this low phosphate paté on Melba toast, toasted bread, or any other cracker, if you're trying to lose weight then go for the low fat cream cheese.

Serves One-Six

- Two spring onions, trimmed and finely sliced

- 200g (7oz) smoked mackerel fillets, skin removed
- One lemon
- One tablespoon creamed horseradish
- Pepper
- 100g (3½oz) cream cheese

Preparation method

1. Break the mackerel into chunks and cut it finely.
2. Add the mackerel, spring onions, cream cheese, creamed horseradish and one lemon zest to a bowl and mix.
3. Squeeze your zested lemon juice into it, and mix again until the paste is coarse.
4. Season with pepper to taste.

Carrot and Coriander Soup

Carrots are a delicious low potassium vegetable, plus the use of a low salt stock ensures that it is kidney friendly. Remember that soup is fluid, so count it if you are on a fluid restriction.

Serves four

- 450g (1lb) carrots, sliced
- Onetbsp of vegetable or olive oil
- One tsp ground coriander
- One onion, sliced
- 1.2 litres/2 pints vegetable stock such as low salt Bouillon
- Large bunch fresh parsley or fresh coriander, roughly chopped (optional)
- One bay leaf
- Freshly ground black pepper

Preparation method

1. In a large pan, heat the oil and add the onions and carrots. Cook for 3-4 minutes before softening begins.
2. Stir in the ground coriander and season properly. One minute to cook.
3. Add the vegetable stock and bay leaf and bring to the boil. Simmer until the vegetables are tender.
4. Remove the bay leaf and use a hand blender or a blender to whizz the soup until smooth. In a clean pan, reheat. Stir in the fresh parsley or coriander and serve with some crusty bread.

Chicken Soup

Making homemade chicken soup is a good way to use up left-over roast chicken, stock, and vegetables. You will want to consider using less fluid at other times if you are fluid-restricted to ensure you don't surpass your restriction. For example, instead of cereal and milk for breakfast, you could have egg on toast, or have a few biscuits with a pudding after a meal instead of custard. We discard the water from the boiled vegetables in this recipe before adding the stock, which helps to reduce the vegetables' potassium content.

Serves Four

- One tbsp of vegetable or olive oil
- Two medium potatoes, peeled
- One litre low salt chicken stock
- One leek
- Three medium carrots
- One tbsp cornflower (if required, see below)
- Squeeze of lemon juice
- Three tbsp Greek yogurt or double cream
- 300g (10½oz) leftover roast chicken, shredded and skin removed

Preparation method

1. Roughly chop the carrots, potatoes, and leek and boil in a large pot of water.
2. Drain the potatoes and vegetables (don't reuse the cooking water), return to the pot and add the stock.
3. Blend the soup with a blender to your preferred consistency.
4. If you want to make your soup thicker: on a low heat, return the pan to the hob, blend the cornflower with a dash of cold water and add to the soup. Stir constantly until the soup thickens when simmering. Add the chicken and leave for five minutes to cook. Add the cream or yogurt and the lemon juice to finish.

Plain Scones

This is a staple recipe that is low in phosphate and potassium and works well as a snack, a pudding, or mall meal. It might sound a lot to make twelve in one go, but they freeze incredibly well-just make sure you use them within one month.

Makes 8-12

- 225g (8oz) self-raising flour
- 150ml milk
- 55g (2oz) butter
- One free-range egg, beaten, to glaze (use a little milk as an alternative)
- 25g (1oz) caster sugar
- pinch of salt

Preparation method

1. Heat the oven to 220°C (200°C Fan)/425°F/Gas 7. Grease a baking sheet lightly.
2. Mix the flour and salt together and rub in the butter.
3. Stir in the sugar, then the milk to get a soft dough.

4. Switch on to a work surface that is floured and knead very gently. Pat it out to a round 2cm/¾in thick. To stamp out rounds, use a 5 cm/2 in cutter and put them on a baking sheet. Lightly knead the remaining dough together and stamp out more scones to use it all up.
5. Use the beaten egg to brush the tops of the scones. Bake until well risen and golden.

Quick and Easy Pancakes

This really is a simple recipe and can be topped with your choice of either savoury or sweet foods.

Serves 2-4

- One egg
- One cup* of milk
- Cooking oil or butter
- One cup* of flour (any type)

* cup = approximately 200ml

Preparation method

1. Place the milk, flour, and egg into a bowl and whisk to mix thoroughly to form a smooth batter.
2. Heat your frying pan untilhot,add the butter or sunflower oil and a large spoonful of the pancake mix.
3. Fry over a medium heat for 10 to 15 minutes until golden brown underneath.
4. Turn the pancake over and cook for a further one-two minutes, or until it is cooked and golden brown.
5. Set this aside and repeat with the remaining batter.

Serving suggestions

Try with tinned pears or stewed apples, peaches, raspberries or strawberries and serve with single cream (remember that tinned fruit is lower in potassium than fresh).

Try serving topped with grated cheese or tuna, ham, or perhaps a hot filling such as chilli for a savoury pancake.

VEGETARIAN DISHES

Cauliflower Cheese

This recipe uses cheese and milk which may mean that it is high in potassium and phosphate; however it makes a large amount of cauliflower cheese to serve four-six people. It should contain 25g/1oz of cheese and 125ml/ ¼ pt milk maximum per portion, which is within the allowances for those requiring restrictions.

Serves four-six

- One large cauliflower (leaves cut off), broken into pieces
- Fourtbsp flour
- 500ml milk
- 100g (3½oz) strong cheddar, grated
- Two-Three tbsp breadcrumbs
- 50g (1¾oz) butter

Preparation method

1. Bring a big saucepan of water to the boil, add the cauliflower and cook for five minutes. Lift a slice to test, it should be cooked. Drain the cauliflower, then pour it into a dish that is ovenproof.
2. Heat the oven to 425 ° F / Gas 7 at 220 ° C (200 ° C fan).
3. Return the saucepan back to the heat and add the flour, butter, and milk. As the butter melts and the mixture comes to the boil, keep whisking quickly-the flour will vanish and the sauce will start thickening. Whisk for two minutes while the sauce bubbles and becomes smooth and thick. Turn the heat off, stir in much of the cheese and dump the cauliflower over it. Scatter over the remaining breadcrumbs and cheese.
4. In the oven, bake the cauliflower cheese for twenty minutes until it bubbles.
   Tip: Make enough for six servings, even if you need less as spare portions can be frozen before being baked.

Pumpkin Risotto

This is a filling meal, and while it contains butternut squash (a vegetable with moderate levels of potassium), it is made with rice (rather than potatoes), which decreases the potassium content of the dish. The cheese used for this recipe is minimal, but you can enjoy this meal without cheese, reducing the phosphate and fat content. Serves 3-4

- 570ml (one pint) vegetable such as low chicken stock or salt Bouillon
- One small onion, chopped
- Twelve fresh sage leaves, chopped finely
- Twotbsp olive oil
- Freshly ground black pepper
- 250g (9oz) pumpkin or butternut squash, diced small ● 50g (2oz) butter

- 170g (6oz) Arborio (risotto) rice
- Piece of vegetarian parmesan-style grating cheese or fresh parmesan (this is optional)

Preparation method

1. Heat the stock and simmer over a very low heat until almost boiling. Sweat the onion in the oil in a separate heavy-based saucepan until soft but not browned. Add the chopped sage and cook.
2. To cover the grains with oil, add the rice and mix well for a few seconds, then pour one-third of the stock in and bring it to a gentle simmer. Cook until it absorbs nearly all the stock. Add the squash or pumpkin and a little more stock, and cook gently until the stock is absorbed.
3. Add the remaining stock until the pumpkin is soft and the rice al dente is sweet. You do not need all the stock, but it should be loose and creamy in texture.
4. Stir the butter into the risotto and add salt and pepper and season well.
5. Add the grated cheese and divide into four servings.

Pastry-less Quiche

This is a very flexible recipe, since rather than the tomatoes, peppers, and mushrooms you can easily substitute all of the vegetables with any of your favorite vegetables, such as peas and dried mint or squash and sage. This dish can be eaten hot or cold as well, making it perfect for home dinner or for a packed lunch. Note that both mushrooms and tomatoes are high potassium foods, but ok when consumed in small amounts.

Serves 4

- One green pepper, diced
- One red pepper, diced
- One onion, chopped
- 75ml milk
- 50g (1¾oz) grated cheddar cheese or use a lower phosphate cheese such as feta
- Eight medium mushrooms, sliced
- 250g (9oz) fat free natural cottage cheese
- Two large or Three medium tomatoes, sliced
- Five eggs

Preparation method

1. Using a small amount of vegetable oil or spray oil to gently fry prepared vegetables (except tomatoes). You still want to make them a little crunchy, so don't overdo the veg.
2. Mix the 5 eggs, 250 g fat-free natural cottage cheese and the milk together-this is not a pretty combination, but stick with it.
3. In an oven-proof flan dish, spread the chopped vegetables out, then pour over the cottage cheese mix.
4. Place the sliced tomatoes on top and sprinkle the cheese on top.

Pop in the oven at 190 ° C (170 ° C fan)/375 ° F / Gas 5, for about thirty to forty-five minutes, or until the quiche is golden brown.

THE VERSATILE MINCE SECTION

- for vegetarians too!!

The entire segment is dedicated to the versatility of mince and contains all kinds of mince: beef pork, chicken, turkey, lamb and vegetarian mince. For each of these recipes, you can decide which mince you'd like to use. It's safer to look for lean or extra lean beef chicken or turkey mince if you're trying to lose weight. Alternatively, you might want to try vegetarian mince, since this is also a good source of protein and naturally low fat.

Kidney Friendly Pasty

These pasties are great served hot from the oven, but in a packed lunch, they are equally tasty cold. In this recipe, we suggest par-boiling the swede and carrot, as this helps lower the potassium content of these vegetables.

Makes approximately six

- One medium carrot, peeled and chopped
- ½ small swede or ¼ large one, peeled and chopped
- 250g (8oz) of your chosen mince
- One medium onion, chopped finely
- Two teaspoons dried parsley
- 120ml low salt stock
- ½ teaspoon of English mustard
- 500g (17oz) ready-made short crust pastry
- Pepper
- One medium egg, lightly whisked

CHAPTER 5

RENAL DIET RECIPES

LIVER OF HEIFER AND ITS ONION COMPOTE

INGREDIENTS

- 1 slice of organic heifer liver
- 2 small onions
- 1 apple Canada
- tablespoon olive oil
- 1 lemon
- 1 slice of cinnamon
- Salt pepper

Instruction

1. Peel and slice the onions. Make them return in half of the olive oil until they become translucent. Salt and pepper them. Cover and cook on very low heat for 30 minutes. Watch for cooking, add a little water if necessary.
2. Wash the lemon under running water, wipe it and squeeze it.
3. Wash the apple, peel it, and remove the fibrous core and seeds. Cut it into cubes — Lemon it to avoid blackening place in a small saucepan with cinnamon and 2 tablespoons water. Cook covered over low heat for 20 minutes. At the end of cooking, crush it in the coarse compote.
4. Cut the liver into strips and cook for 2 to 3 minutes in the pan with the remaining olive oil. Once cooked, mix it with the onion compote.
5. Enjoy it immediately, accompanied by the applesauce.

Nutritional fact

Thanks to the liver, this dish is very rich in iron and zinc, easily assimilated, trace elements essential for the proper functioning of the immune system. It may be particularly recommended for young children, regulated women, and endurance athletes, who often lack iron.

In case of excess cholesterol, do not consume more than one shot per week.

PALETTE OF PORK AND ITS VEGETABLES

INGREDIENTS

- 1 pallet of bone-in pork of 1 kilo
- 100 g smoked diced bacon
- 1/4 green cabbage

- 300 g carrots
- 200 g turnips
- 400 g of firm-fleshed potatoes type BF 15
- 2 onions
- 2 cloves
- 1 bouquet garni
- 1 tablet of organic vegetable broth
- Salt pepper

Instruction

1. Place the bacon in a saute pan and sauté over medium heat, stirring. Add the palette and use the fat rendered to brown the meat, about 5 minutes on each side. Add a peeled onion and chopped, also brown. Add 1/2 litre of water, the bouquet garni, and the second onion stuck cloves and the crumbled broth.
2. Wash the piece of cabbage, remove the outer leaves too hard, and its core. Dip it in a pan of boiling salted water and let it whiten for 10 minutes. Drain it and cut it into strips. Add it to the sauté pan with the palette, salt, and pepper it, continue cooking for 15 minutes.
3. Wash and peel carrots, turnips, and potatoes. Cut them into slices. Add the carrots and turnips in the pan, salt, and pepper. Continue cooking for 10 minutes. Add the potatoes and finish cooking for 20 minutes. Rectify the seasoning, remove the bouquet garni and onion pique clove.

Nutritional fact

This complete dish simultaneously brings functional meat proteins, fibre, and vitamins from vegetables, energy carbohydrates from potatoes. Low fat, it is suitable for overweight (450 kcal per serving). For a balanced meal, add milk and seasonal fruit.

EXOTIC FRUIT VERRINES

INGREDIENTS

- 2 kiwis
- 1 mango
- 1/2 grenade
- 1/4 litre of semi-skimmed milk
- 2 eggs
- 25 g of sugar
- 1 vanilla pod
- 2 half-sheets of gelatin or 1/2 teaspoon of agar agar

Instruction

1. Wash the vanilla pod, slice it in half, and place it in a saucepan with the milk. Heat and stop the fire just before boiling. Let the vanilla steep in the milk.
2. Position the gelatin in a bowl of cold water.
3. Separate the whites and egg yolks. Whip the yolks with the sugar. Add the cooled and filtered milk. Pour everything into the saucepan and cook on low heat, constantly stirring until the cream thickens. Add

drained half-leaves of gelatin or agar-agar, wait for their perfect dissolution to cut the fire. Divide the custard into four glasses and refrigerate for at least 2 hours.
4. Wash the fruits under running water and sponge them out. Peel the kiwis and mango and cut them into cubes. Collect the grains from the pomegranate. Mix these fruits gently and divide them into the glasses. Enjoy it immediately.

Nutritional interest

Thanks to exotic fruits, these verrines are rich in antioxidant vitamins: beta-carotene, vitamins B9, and C, which help the body defend itself against infections.

To balance your menu, consume a verrine at the end of a meal with vegetables, meat, fish or legumes, and starchy foods.

CHICKPEA SALAD

INGREDIENTS

- 150 g chickpeas
- 1 onion
- 1 clove
- 1 clove of garlic
- 1 bouquet garni
- 200 g celery-branch
- 1 lemon
- 5 tablespoons of olive oil
- 1 tip of curry
- 1 tablespoon chopped chives
- Salt pepper

INSTRUCTION

1. Position the chickpeas in a large bowl filled with cold water and let them soak for 12 hours.
2. Peel the onion and garlic. Drain the chickpeas. Place them in a casserole with 1/2 litre of cold water, the bouquet garni, and the onion stuck clove, the clove of garlic, some grains of pepper. Cover, cook for 2 hours.
3. Wash the celery, detach its branches from the bulb, remove the top of the leaves, detail it in the sticks.
4. Wash the lemon and squeeze its juice — mix 2 tablespoons with the olive oil and the curry.
5. Drain the chickpeas well. Mix with celery. Add salt and pepper. Season with the olive oil vinaigrette and add the chives.

Nutritional fact

This salad, rich in fibre and protein (chickpeas) is very satiating and has a low glycemic index. It can be especially recommended in case of diabetes. Calorie intake reasonable 250 kcal per serving. It is suitable for overweight.

The consumption of pulses is recommended at least twice a week, in order to increase vegetable protein and reduce animal protein.

ROQUEFORT PEAR TOAST

INGREDIENTS

- 8 slices of walnut bread (120 g)
- 1 jar of 100 g of white cheese with 3% fat
- 60 g of Roquefort cheese
- 2 ripe Williams or Guyot pears
- 1 lemon
- 4 nuts

INSTRUCTIONS

1. Toast the slices of bread.
2. Remove the nuts from their shells.
3. Mix together the cottage cheese and Roquefort cheese. Spread toast with this mixture.
4. Wash the lemon, sponge it, and squeeze its juice.
5. Wash the pears, peel them, remove their central part and their pips, divide them into tiny dice. Lemon immediately to prevent the pears from turning black.
6. Spread the pears over the toasts. Add a walnut kernel per toast.

Nutritional fact

Made from walnut bread, Roquefort pear toasts provide 25% of the recommended daily intake of omega 3 essential fats, which are beneficial for cardiovascular prevention. They are rich in fibre (bread, pear, nuts), satiating, and regulating the transit.

Spread with lean fresh cheese with 3% fat and a small amount of Roquefort, they are suitable for hypercholesterolemia.

Whether you eat them as a starter or as an appetizer, you can balance your meal by moderating starchy foods and preparing vegetables.

SHORTBREAD WITH JAM

INGREDIENTS

- 100 g of wheat flour type 55
- 50 g butter or margarine rich in omega 3 not lightened
- 50 g of sugar
- 1 egg
- 120 g of strawberry or apricot jam, homemade if possible
- 2 tablespoons icing sugar
- 1 large star-shaped cookie cutter
- 1 round-shaped cookie cutter 1.5 cm in diameter

INSTRUCTIONS

1. Separate the whites from the egg yolk.
2. In a bowl, mix the flour, sugar, and butter until you have a texture of sand. Add the egg yolk to mix the dough ball. Let the dough rest in the refrigerator for at least 30 minutes.
3. Preheat the oven to 180 ° C. Arrange a sheet of baking paper on a baking sheet.
4. Spread the dough. Cut star-shaped shortbread. In half of these shortbreads, cut a small circle of dough in the middle.
5. Arrange the shortbread on the plate and bake for 15 minutes.
6. Let the shortbread a little cool. Cover each shortbread with jam and sprinkle each shortbread with icing sugar. Arrange the shortbreads pierced over jammed biscuits.

Nutritional fact

Made with flour and jam, these biscuits are rich in carbohydrates and energy. They have their place at the end of a meal without starch or snack after a light lunch. They can also be used as a snack, in recovery after a sports training.

Low in fat, they are suitable for hypercholesterolemia.

SKEWERS OF SEITAN

INGREDIENTS

- 1 block of seitan 240 g
- 1 lemon
- 3 tablespoons sesame oil
- 2 onions
- 1 clove of garlic
- 1 tablespoon acacia honey
- 1 tablespoon paprika
- 200 g cherry tomatoes
- 100 g of Paris mushrooms
- 2 tablespoons sesame seeds
- Salt pepper

INSTRUCTIONS

1. Wash the lemon under running water, sponge it, and squeeze it.
2. Peel the onions, slice them. Peel and slice the clove of garlic.
3. Cut the seitan into cubes.
4. Mix honey and lemon juice, add oil and paprika, salt, and pepper. Arrange the seitan, onions, and garlic in a dish and sprinkle with the marinade. Allow in the refrigerator for at least 1 hour.
5. Wash the tomatoes and mushrooms, sponge them out. Cut the mushrooms into strips.
6. Make skewers by alternating seitan cubes with onion rings, cherry tomatoes, and mushroom slices. Filter the marinade.
7. Cook the kebabs on a pan in their marinade, 2 min 30 on each side over medium heat. Drain them and roll them in the sesame seeds. Iron for 1 min in the pan, just time to lightly brown the sesame seeds.

Nutritional fact

These skewers provide as much protein as a small steak, the quality of which can be optimized by combining legume proteins, such as lentils. With a reasonable energy intake of 280 kcal, they are suitable for overweight.

BEAN SALAD TO SHELL

INGREDIENTS

- 150 g of shelling beans
- 30 g pasta, farfalle type
- 150 g fresh green beans
- 200 g tomatoes
- 1 carrot
- 1 bouquet garni
- 4 tablespoons olive oil
- 2 tablespoons balsamic vinegar
- 1/2 teaspoon of mustard
- 1 shallot
- 2 teaspoons chopped parsley
- 1 teaspoon chopped basil
- Salt pepper

INSTRUCTIONS

1. Shell the beans. Position them in a large saucepan and cover them completely with cold water. Add the bouquet garni, cover the pan. Let it simmer for 35 minutes.
2. Wash the green beans and mop them up. Cut in half, salt, and steam for 15 minutes.
3. Cook the pasta the time indicated on the package.
4. Peel and chop the shallot.
5. Prepare the vinaigrette with oil, vinegar, mustard, salt, and pepper. Add the shallot.
6. Wash tomatoes and carrot under running water. Rind off and grate the carrot, cut the tomatoes into wedges.
7. In a salad bowl, combine the shelling beans and the drained pasta, the green beans, the tomatoes, the carrot, and the herbs. Add the vinaigrette and mix gently. Correct the seasoning if necessary.

Nutritional fact

This salad is rich in fibre and antioxidants: vitamin E, vitamin C, lycopene (tomatoes), beta-carotene (carrot). It combines the complementary proteins of beans to shelling and pasta. By doubling the proportions, you will get a balanced vegetarian main course.

Raspberry tartlets without gluten

INGREDIENTS

- 100 g of rice flour
- 30 g of almond powder
- 30 g butter or margarine rich in omega 3 not lightened
- 90 g of sugar
- 2 eggs
- 20 g of cornflower
- 25 cl of semi-skimmed milk
- 1 vanilla pod
- 500 g raspberries
- 1 tablespoon icing sugar

INSTRUCTIONS

1. Heat the milk until boiling. Cut the fire. Split the vanilla pod in half and let it steep in the milk.
2. Mix the rice flour with the almond powder and 60 g sugar. Add the melted butter and work the dough with a fork until you get a sandy texture. Combine the dough with 1 beaten egg and refrigerate for at least 30 minutes.
3. Separate the white and yellow from the remaining egg. Whip the yolk with 30 g of sugar. Add the cornflower, then the milk, previously filtered, very gradually. Cook this cream over low heat, constantly stirring until thickened (about 3 minutes).
4. Preheat the oven to 180 ° C. Spread the pie dough and divide it into four lightly greased tart pans. Cover each tart with parchment paper and dried vegetables — Cook the tarts for 25 minutes.
5. Wash the raspberries under a stream of running water. Sponge them carefully and remove their peduncles.
6. Wait until the tartlets are cold to garnish with pastry cream and raspberries. Sprinkle with icing sugar.

Nutritional fact

Made from rice flour and corn, this tart is suitable for gluten intolerance. Thanks to raspberries, it is a good source of fibre and vitamin C. Energetic; it has its place at the end of a meal without starchy foods.

Quiche with ratatouille

INGREDIENTS

- 250g of flour
- 125 g butter or margarine rich in omega 3 not lightened
- 2 zucchini
- 1 eggplant
- 3 tomatoes
- 1 yellow pepper
- 1 onion
- 2 tablespoons olive oil
- 1 bouquet garni
- 4 eggs
- 100 g grated Emmental cheese
- Salt pepper

INSTRUCTIONS

1. In a small salad bowl, mix the flour and butter until you have a texture of sand. Add a little salt water to combine the ball of dough. Let stand in the refrigerator for at least 30 minutes.
2. Peel and slice the onion. Wash the vegetables. Peel the zucchini and cut into slices. Cut the eggplant into cubes. Remove the peduncle, seeds and whitish fibrous parts of pepper, cut into strips.
3. Fry the onion with the olive oil in a frying pan. Add pepper, zucchini, and eggplant, brown while stirring. Add the tomatoes, the bouquet garni, salt, and pepper. Cover; simmer on low heat for 20-30 minutes. At the end of cooking, discover to let evaporate the water of constitution of vegetables.
4. Preheat the oven to 200-210 ° C. Spread the dough and place it in a pie dish. Cover with parchment paper and dried vegetables — Cook for 20 minutes.
5. Mix the well-reduced ratatouille with the eggs and Emmental cheese. Pour this mixture onto the pie shell, free of parchment paper. Finish cooking in the oven for 15 minutes.

Nutritional fact

The ratatouille quiche is a complete balanced dish, which can be supplemented with dairy and fresh fruit.

Zucchini/shrimp verrines

INGREDIENTS

- 2 zucchini
- 2 shallots
- 2 tablespoons olive oil
- 1/4 teaspoon of curry
- 100 g shelled shrimp
- 1 bunch of chervil
- Salt pepper

INSTRUCTION

1. Peel and mince the shallots.
2. Wash the zucchini, sponge them, peel them, and cut them in small dice.
3. Place the oil in a pan with the curry. Add the shallots and zucchini to make them come back. Add salt and pepper. Cover, cook for 15-20 minutes over low heat. At the end of cooking, if necessary, evaporate the vegetable water.
4. Divide the zucchini fondue into 4 verrines. Add the shrimp on top and decorate with chervil sprigs.

Nutritional fact

Made from ingredients from the Mediterranean diet, this verrine provides multiple antioxidants (vitamins C and E, beta-carotene, polyphenols, and selenium) to protect the health. Very low fat and low in calories (100 kcal per serving), it is particularly suitable for hypercholesterolemia or overweight.

Homemade sauerkraut

INGREDIENTS

- 1 white cabbage, preferably organic
- 2 teaspoons of salt
- 1 teaspoon juniper berries
- 1 teaspoon of peppercorns
- 6 bay leaves
- 2 glass jars of 1 liter with a screw lid

INSTRUCTION

1. Wash the jars and their lid thoroughly.
2. Put away the outer leaves and the core of the cabbage. Cut it into skinny strips.
3. In each jar, alternate layers of cabbage, each with salt, juniper berries, peppercorns, and bay leaves. Pack well.
4. If there is a bit of room at the top of the jar, add water that has been boiled and chilled. Close the jars without screwing them in completely.
5. Leave the jars at room temperature for 2 days, so that the cabbage can ferment. Then, screw them thoroughly and place them in the refrigerator for 1 month before eating. You can keep them for up to 6 months. Once started, consume them within 48 hours.

Nutritional fact

Preparing homemade sauerkraut helps to consume raw. And so, to enjoy more of its vitamins (C and B9 in particular) and natural lactic ferments at the origin of its obtaining. Some of these ferments reach the colon alive and contribute to the functional diversity of the microbiota (intestinal flora), favorable to health.

Namely: 100 g of sauerkraut provides 100% of the daily need for vitamin K, a contribution that must be taken into account by people on anticoagulant therapy.

Homemade yogurts with a pressure cooker

INGREDIENTS

- 90cl of semi-skimmed UHT milk
- 1 jar of plain yogurt with whole commercial milk
- 4 tablespoons of skimmed milk powder
- 1 organic orange
- 1 cooking thermometer

INSTRUCTIONS

1. Wash the orange under running water, sponge it with absorbent paper and recover its zest.
2. Place the milk and orange zest in a saucepan, heat to a boil. Then, turn off the heat and let the zest infuse until the milk temperature drops to 45 ° C (check with the thermometer).
3. During this time, fill the pressure cooker with water for one third. Close the lid and put it on the fire. Leave several minutes under pressure. Then, cut the fire and let the steam escape.
4. Sift the milk through the sieve to remove the orange zest. Whisk it with yogurt and milk powder. Divide into 8 glass yogurt jars.
5. Discard the boiling water from the pressure cooker. Place the pots in the basket of the casserole and enclose them immediately in the still very hot casserole. Let it ferment at room temperature for 4 - 5 hours. Then place the yogurt in the refrigerator.

Nutritional fact

Yogurt makes it possible to take advantage of the good proteins and the calcium of the milk, even in case of intolerance to lactose (sugar of cow, goat, and sheep milk), that its lactic ferments have the capacity to digest. It can be called probiotic, because its regular consumption contributes to the development, within the microbiota (intestinal flora), of bacteria considered as beneficial to health.

Omelet with chicken livers

INGREDIENTS

- 6 eggs
- 150 g of chicken livers
- 2 shallots
- 3 tablespoons of olive oil
- 1 tsp chopped parsley, 1 teaspoon chopped chives, 1 tsp chopped tarragon
- Salt pepper

INSTRUCTIONS

1. Pare and cut in 4 the chicken livers. Peel and mince the shallots.
2. Fry the chicken livers in the olive oil and cook for 3 to 4 minutes. Then, reserve them and sweat the shallots over a fairly soft fire. Mix them with the livers and reserve.
3. Beat the eggs, salt and pepper them. Cook them in a sloppy omelet. Spread over the chicken livers and herbs.
4. Fold the omelet and slide it onto a serving dish.

Nutritional fact

Poultry liver omelet provides good protein that is effective for growing children, as well as maintaining muscle mass in adults. It is a good source of vitamin D: 2g per serving, or 40% of the recommended daily intake.

Its reasonable caloric intake (225 kcal) allows us to consume it in case of overweight.

To know: this recipe is not recommended for pregnant women and children under 3 years because of the very high vitamin A content of chicken livers.

Cheesecake

INGREDIENTS

- 350 g of 3% fat (3% fat) white cheese enriched with vitamin D (Calin + type)
- 2 eggs
- 35 g of Maïzena ®
- 60 g of sugar
- 1 teaspoon of bitter almond extract
- 1 tablespoon flaked almonds
- Salt

INSTRUCTIONS

1. Preheat the oven to 170 ° C. Garnish a mold to run out of baking paper.
2. Separate the yolks and whites from the eggs. Climb these in very firm snow with a pinch of salt.
3. Mix the Maïzena® gradually with the cottage cheese. Then add the egg yolks, the sugar, then the almond extract. When the preparation is homogeneous, gently add the egg whites.
4. Pour the dough into the mold and bake for 40 to 45 minutes. Check the cooking by pricking the cake with a knife tip. Wait until it has cooled down to remove the baking paper.
5. Pass the almonds quickly in a non-stick frying pan for browning. Decorate the cake.

Nutritional fact

The cottage cheesecake provides good protein (cottage cheese, egg), as well as energy carbohydrates (sugar, Maizena). Made from white cheese enriched with calcium and vitamin D, it provides respectively 25 and 100% of the recommended daily intake to an adult in these micronutrients. It may be particularly recommended for growing teenagers and seniors for the prevention of osteoporosis.

Pear and walnut

INGREDIENTS

- 1 beautiful pear
- 80 g of butter
- 1/2 teaspoon of vanilla extract
- 2 eggs
- 100 g of sugar
- 50 g of chestnut flour
- 50 g of wheat flour type 55
- 1/2 sachet of yeast
- 80 g unsweetened cocoa powder
- 14 nuts
- 2 teaspoons icing sugar

INSTRUCTIONS

1. Preheat the oven to 180 - 200 ° C. Lightly grease a non-stick mold with an oiled brush.
2. Wash the pear, peel it, remove its central part and its seeds, cut it in big quarters. Put it in the pan with 20 g of butter and vanilla. Remove it from the fire as soon as it begins to caramelize. Arrange it at the bottom of the mold.
3. Schell nuts.
4. Separate the whites from the egg yolks. Beat the egg whites with a pinch of salt.
5. Mix the egg yolks with the sugar. Add the remaining 60 g of butter. Gradually add the two flours with the yeast, then the cocoa powder, and finally 12 nuts. Carefully incorporate the whites into the snow.
6. Pour the mix into the pan over the pear and bake for 25 minutes at 180 ° C. Check the cooking with a knife tip (the dough does not stick when the cake is cooked).
7. Unmount the pound. Sprinkle with icing sugar and decorate with the remaining 2 nuts

Potato salad with smoked herring

INGREDIENTS

- 400 g of firm-fleshed potatoes such as Amandine or Belle de Fontenay
- 1 small beet
- 2 shallots
- 150 g sweet smoked herring fillets
- 4 tablespoons ISIO 4 mixed oil
- 2 tablespoons vinegar
- 1 teaspoon of mustard
- 2 teaspoons chopped dill (fresh or frozen)
- Salt pepper

INSTRUCTIONS

1. Wash the potatoes under running water, peel them, slice them and steam them for 20 minutes.
2. Cut the herring into cubes.
3. Peel the beetroot and cut into cubes. Peel and slice the shallots
4. Mix mustard, oil, vinegar, and shallots.
5. Divide the still-warm potatoes and beet into 4 serving plates: salt very lightly and pepper. Add herring and vinaigrette, sprinkle with dill. Taste immediately

Nutritional fact

This salad is rich in protein (herring), as well as in fiber and complex carbohydrates (potato). But, his main interests are his contributions of essential omega 3 and vitamin D, abundant in oil ISIO 4 and herring. One serving provides about 12 grams of vitamin D, more than double the recommended daily intake.

This salad is suitable for diabetes or overweight (250 kcal per person), provided it is consumed within a balanced meal, combined with a good vegetable dish, a dairy, and fresh seasonal fruit.

Salmon with lentils

INGREDIENTS

- 1 salmon steak
- 50 g du Puy lentils
- 1 carrot
- 1 onion
- 1 bouquet garni
- 1 small white leek
- 1 teaspoon dried tomatoes
- 1 shallot
- 1 tablespoon olive oil
- 1 tablespoon dry white wine
- Salt and pepper

INSTRUCTIONS

1. Wash the carrot and peel it. Peel the onion. Cut these vegetables into large slices. Place them with the lentils and the bouquet garni in a saucepan. Cover with cold water, cover, and cook for 30 minutes in small broths. Salt at the end of cooking and remove bouquet garni and slices of vegetables.
2. Wash the leek and thinly slice it. Peel and chop the shallot. Sweat these vegetables with olive oil. Then add the white wine and 2 tablespoons water, cover, cook on low heat for 20 minutes. Add the dried tomatoes, a little water if necessary, and finish cooking 10 min.
3. Steam the salmon for 10 minutes.
4. Arrange salmon and lentils on a serving platter. Spread over the leek fondue.

Nutritional fact

Very rich in proteins (salmon, lentils) and fiber (lentils, vegetables), this main course is particularly satisfying. Associated with a dairy and a fruit, it allows us to "hold" without hunger until the next meal and so not to nibble. It is particularly suitable for diabetes or overweight (510 kcal per serving).

Spinach egg cake

INGREDIENTS

- 1 commercial buckwheat pancake
- 150 g spinach
- 1 egg
- 1 tablespoon of olive oil
- 1 teaspoon chopped parsley
- Salt pepper

INSTRUCTIONS

1. Wash the spinach under running water with a strainer. Drain them in a dishcloth or salad spinner. Remove their tail and ribs if necessary. Place in a pan with olive oil, salt, and pepper. Let them cook for 5 minutes on high heat, just until their water evaporates. Reserve them.
2. Place the pancake in the pan so that it warms up. Garnish with spinach. Break the egg over the center, salt, and pepper. As soon as the white is cooked, remove the pan from the heat.
3. Sprinkle with parsley and fold the 4 corners of the cake. Enjoy it immediately.

Nutritional fact

The egg whip spinach is a complete dish, which simultaneously provides good protein (egg), energy complex carbohydrates (buckwheat), and vegetables. Thanks to spinach, it is particularly rich in beta-carotene (100% of the recommended daily intake of an adult), vitamins C and B9 (50% of the recommended intake). It also provides a quarter of the daily needs of fiber and calcium.

Not very fat, it has a reasonable energy intake: 290 kcal, it is suitable for overweight.

In cases of high cholesterol, remember to count the egg in your weekly quota.

Cups of strawberries with mango

INGREDIENTS

- 400 g strawberries
- 1 mango
- 60 g frozen blackcurrant kernels
- 2 teaspoons honey all flowers
- 4 tablespoons of homemade pressed orange juice or fresh ray
- 1 tablespoon of silver-colored sugar pearls
- 4 lace pancakes

INSTRUCTIONS

1. A few hours in advance, place the black currants in the refrigerator to thaw.
2. Wash the strawberries under running water, pat them well with paper towels and shake them off. Wash the mango under running water and sponge it.
3. Mix the honey with the orange juice.
4. Cut the mango in half (cut flush with the core). Peel each half and cut into cubes. Cut the strawberries in half. Delicately mix mango, strawberries, blackcurrant, and orange sauce. Divide the fruit salad into 4 cups. Garnish with sugar pearls and arrange a lace crepe in each cup. Enjoy it immediately.

Nutritional fact

The strawberry mango cut combines 4 fruits richest in vitamin C so that a serving represents 80% of the recommended daily intake to an adult. It is also a healthy source of beta-carotene (especially thanks to mango), vitamin B9, and fiber: 15% of the recommended intake for each of these nutrients.

Providing potassium and simple sugars, based on fruits with alkalizing virtues, it can be offered in recovery after an effort to children or adult athletes.

Coconut-pineapple mousse

INGREDIENTS

- 3 eggs
- 37.5 cl of coconut milk
- 60 g of sugar
- 1/4 to 1/3 pineapple (200 g net)
- 5 half-sheets of gelatin
- 1 pinch of salt

INSTRUCTIONS

1. Separate the yolks and egg whites.
2. Soak the gelatin in a bowl of cold water.
3. Whip the egg yolks with the sugar. Gradually add the coconut milk. Put everything into a saucepan and cook on low heat, constantly stirring until the cream is tableclothed.
4. Drain the gelatin carefully and add it to the coconut cream. Whip, and as soon as the gelatin is dissolved, remove the pan from the heat. Let cool for 1 hour in the refrigerator.
5. Peel the pineapple: remove its skin. It's the central hard part and its "eyes." Make sure you have 200 g of flesh that you cut into small cubes.
6. Add a pinch of salt to the egg whites and beat in the snow firmly. Mix them gently with the coconut cream. Add the pineapple dice. Divide the mousse into 4 ramekins and put in at least 2 hours in the refrigerator before eating.

Nutritional fact

Thanks to coconut milk, the coconut-pineapple mousse is rich in potassium, vegetable iron, and vitamin B5. Thanks to the eggs, it provides proteins of excellent nutritional quality. Coconut milk is good and high in saturated fat (17%), but it is mainly lauric acid, which, according to recent studies, does not affect the blood cholesterol level.

Spinach gratin with goat cheese

INGREDIENTS

- 250 g fresh spinach
- 1 teaspoon of butter (10 g)
- 1 teaspoon flour (10 g)
- 10 cl of goat's milk
- 30 g fresh goat cheese
- Nutmeg
- Salt pepper

INSTRUCTION

1. Wash the spinach under running water, sponge them out, mop them up. Place them in a pan with salt and pepper, cover, cook on low heat for 15 minutes.
2. Preheat the oven to 200 ° C.
3. Place the butter and sifted the flour in a saucepan. Mix over low heat. Add the milk gradually. Salt and pepper, grate some nutmeg. Cook over low heat, constantly stirring for some minutes.
4. Mix the bechamel with the well-drained spinach. Arrange everything in an individual gratin dish Emit the goat cheese over it — Bake in the oven for about some minutes.

Nutritional fact

Thanks to spinach, this gratin is rich in vegetable iron, vitamins E and K, anti-oxidant carotenoids, and fiber. Enriched with milk and goat cheese, it provides nearly 400 mg of calcium or 45% of the recommended daily intake to an adult. This dish is particularly suitable for children, teenagers, pregnant women (if you choose a cheese made from pasteurized milk), and the elderly.

Eggs with milk and goat cheese

INGREDIENTS

- 2 eggs
- 40 cl whole goat's milk
- 60 g Pouligny-Saint-Pierre (goat cheese)
- 2 slices of Bayonne ham (60 g)
- Pepper

INSTRUCTIONS

1. Preheat the oven to 180 ° C.
2. Cut the cheese into small cubes. Slice the ham in chiffonade.
3. Beat the eggs in an omelet. Add the milk gradually. Add the diced goat cheese, ham, and a little pepper.
4. Divide the resulting preparation into four individual ramekins. Arrange the ramekins in an oven dish in which you have poured the bottom of the water so that the milk eggs cook in a bain-marie.
5. Bake for 30 minutes at 180 ° C. Check the cooking of the eggs with a knife tip (the preparation does not stick when the eggs are cooked).

Nutritional fact

Milk and goat eggs are rich in high-quality protein for growth as well as muscle maintenance. Can be served as a main dish, replacing the meat.

Thanks to milk and goat cheese, they provide vitamins B2, B12, A, and D, as well as calcium: 150 mg per serving, or 17% of the recommended daily intake.

They are especially suitable for children, teens, athletes, and the elderly.

Palets with squash seeds

INGREDIENTS

- 80 g flour type 55 or 80
- 5 tablespoons of olive oil
- 1/2 teaspoon of baking soda (yeast)
- 40 g squash seeds
- 30 g dried tomatoes
- 1 teaspoon dried oregano
- Salt

INSTRUCTIONS

1. Mix the flour, baking soda, squash seeds, sun-dried tomatoes, and oregano. Include 4 tablespoons of olive oil and 1 pinch of salt. Add a few spoons of water to form a ball of dough. Let stand at least 30 minutes at room temperature.
2. Preheat the oven to 180 ° C. Arrange a sheet of baking paper on a baking sheet. Brush with the remaining oil.
3. Sprinkle with flour the work plan. Roll out the dough as finely as possible with a rolling pin. Use a cookie cutter to cut pucks. Arrange the pucks on the parchment paper. Bake for 15 minutes at 185 ° C. Check the cooking with a knife tip (the dough does not stick when the puck is cooked).

Nutritional fact

The squash seeds combine healthy ingredients, useful in cardiovascular prevention: olive oil and squash seeds, high in unsaturated fats that help reduce the level of bad blood cholesterol and tomatoes, including lycopene (which colors them in red) is a powerful antioxidant.

In case of diabetes, know that a portion of these pucks corresponds to 30 g of bread.

Whiting bread with sesame

INGREDIENT

- 400 g whiting fillets
- 4 tablespoons sesame oil
- 1 lemon
- 1 tablespoon soy sauce
- 1 clove of garlic
- 2 tablespoons minced lemongrass
- 1 small piece of ginger 1 cm
- 4 tablespoons sesame seeds
- 2 eggs
- Salt pepper

INSTRUCTIONS

1. Wash the lemon under running water, sponge it, squeeze it. Peel and slice the clove of garlic. Pass the ginger under the water, sponge it, grate it.
2. Prepare a marinade with 2 tablespoons of sesame oil, lemon juice, soy sauce, lemongrass, garlic, ginger, and a little pepper. Arrange the whiting fillets in the marinade and reserve them in the refrigerator for 2 hours.
3. Then very carefully drain the fish fillets. Cook them for 5 minutes, steaming.
4. Separate the egg whites from the yolks. Spread each fillet of whiting in the egg yolk and then in the sesame seeds to form a breadcrumb. Salt slightly. Quickly pass the breaded fish fillets in a non-stick frying pan with the remaining 2 spoons of oil. As soon as the sesame seeds are golden brown, stop cooking. Enjoy it immediately.

Nutritional fact

Whiting is rich in protein of excellent quality for growth, as is the maintenance of muscle mass. Breaded with sesame, it is also an excellent source of calcium, magnesium, and iron. It is suitable for hypercholesterolemia since sesame provides mainly unsaturated fats.

Almond/Pear Express Cream

INGREDIENTS

- 1 pot of semi-skimmed milk cheese with 3% fat
- 1 teaspoon of almond powder
- 1/2 teaspoon of flax seeds
- 2 drops of bitter almond extract
- 1 teaspoon of honey
- 1 lemon
- 1 pear
- 1 small square of dark chocolate

INSTRUCTIONS

1. Place the flax seeds in a non-stick pan. Roast them for 2 minutes over medium heat, stirring them, so they do not burn.
2. Wash the lemon under running water, sponge it, and squeeze it.
3. Mix the white cheese with almond powder, bitter almond extract, 2 teaspoons lemon juice, honey, and flax seeds.
4. Wash the pear, peel it, dice it, and lemon it. Mix with almond cream.
5. Slice the chocolate into thin chips and sprinkle the cream. Enjoy it immediately.

Nutritional fact

The almond/pear cream is a good source of calcium, particularly recommended for growing young people or seniors in the prevention of osteoporosis. Rich in fiber, it is satisfying and useful to regularise the transit. Thanks to flaxseed, it provides 50% of the recommended daily intake of essential Omega 3. As almonds mainly provide monounsaturated fats (the same as in olive oil), it can be supported in cases of hypercholesterolemia.

Seasonal vegetable cake

INGREDIENTS

- 100 g of flour type 55
- 2 eggs
- 3 tablespoons of olive oil
- 300 g of already cooked vegetables: carrots, cauliflower, zucchini, broccoli, spinach, peas ...
- 80 ml of semi-skimmed milk
- 1/2 sachet of yeast
- 40 g of goat cheese
- 40 g of Emmentaler
- 1 teaspoon chopped parsley
- 1 teaspoon chopped mint
- Salt pepper

INSTRUCTIONS

1. Heat the oven to 200 ° C. Line a small cake tin with parchment paper.
2. Quickly pass the vegetables in the pan with 1 spoon of oil to lightly grill. Season them with the herbs.
3. Mix the flour with the yeast, then the eggs. Gradually add the milk and the remaining 2 spoons of oil. Add salt and pepper. Finish by incorporating vegetables, diced goat cheese, and grated Emmental cheese.
4. Pour the mix into the cake pan and bake for 30 minutes. Check the cooking with a knife tip (when the cake is cooked, the dough does not stick to the knife).

Nutritional fact

The seasonal vegetable cake is an energy starter rich in complex carbohydrates and protein.

In case of diabetes, one serving replaces 40 g of bread (1/6 of baguette) or 100 g of starch (3 tablespoons). In the case of hypercholesterolemia, avoid consuming other cheese during the day.

ZUCCHINI FLAN

INGREDIENTS

- 1 zucchini
- 1 tomato
- 1 shallot
- 1 teaspoon of olive oil
- 1 pinch of oregano
- 1 egg
- 2 tablespoons cottage cheese
- 1 tablespoon thick cream
- 1 teaspoon Maïzena
- 1 tablespoon grated Emmental cheese
- Salt pepper

INSTRUCTIONS

1. Wash the zucchini and tomato under running water, pat them and peel them. Remove the fibrous central part of the tomato and cut it into quarters. Cut the zucchini into thin slices.
2. Peel and chop the shallot. Sweat over fairly low heat in olive oil for a few minutes, then add the zucchini and tomato. Add salt, pepper, and oregano, cover and cook for 15 minutes on low heat. At the end of cooking, discover the vegetables to reduce them well.
3. Preheat the oven to 180 ° C. Beat the omelet egg and mix it with the Fromage blanc, the cream, and the Maïzena. Add salt and pepper.
4. Place the vegetables in the bottom of an individual gratin dish. Cover them with gratin and sprinkle with grated cheese — Bake for 15 minutes at 180 ° C.

Nutritional fact

The zucchini custard is a complete dish, which can be combined with a slice of bread and fruit for a balanced meal.

It helps to provide good protein (egg, cottage cheese, Emmental) to those who have difficulty in eating meat, including the elderly.

MUSHROOM CAKE AO-NORI

INGREDIENTS

- 80 g of buckwheat flour
- 5 eggs
- 600 g mushrooms from Paris
- 2 shallots
- 2 cloves garlic
- 2 tablespoons olive oil
- 40 g of ao-nori (green algae) in the jar
- 1 tablespoon chopped parsley
- 1 tablespoon of sunflower oil
- Salt pepper

INSTRUCTIONS

1. Prepare the dough by mixing the buckwheat flour with 20 cl of water, a nice pinch of salt, and 1/4 egg beaten into an omelet. Cover the salad bowl and let the dough rest in the refrigerator for 1 hour.
2. Drain and slice the ao-nori. Peel and slice garlic and shallots. Wash the mushrooms under running water, remove their earthy foot, cut them into slices. In a pan, sauté garlic, shallots, and mushrooms with olive oil. Salt and pepper, sprinkle with ao-nori. Cook for 10 minutes (all the mushrooms water must be evaporated) and add the parsley.
3. Bake 4 patties in a lightly greased non-stick pan with an oiled brush.
4. Spread the pan-fried mushrooms on 4 patties. Iron each pancake in the pan. Break an egg in the center. Once the white is cooked, fold the edges of the cake to give it a square shape and serve it immediately.

Nutritional fact

The mushroom cake ao-nori is a complete dish: it provides complex energy carbohydrates (flour), proteins (eggs), and fiber (mushrooms, algae). Thanks to the ao-nori, it is a good source of iron and iodine.

Its energy intake is reasonable: 280 kcal per galette. It can be consumed in case of the celiac disease since buckwheat does not contain gluten

VEGETABLE TOAST

INGREDIENTS

- 30 g chickpeas
- 1 big tomato "Heart of beef" (200 to 250 g)
- 30 g red pepper
- 1 clove of garlic
- 1 teaspoon chopped parsley
- 3 teaspoons of olive oil
- 1/2 teaspoon chopped basil
- 1 nice slice of country bread (50 to 60 g)
- Salt pepper

INSTRUCTIONS

1. Soak the chickpeas in cold water for an hour. The next day, drain them carefully and allow them to dry thoroughly before cooking.
2. Peel the garlic. Wash the piece of pepper, remove its whitish fibrous parts and seeds. Wash the tomato, remove the fibrous central part.
3. Mix together the chickpeas, the clove of garlic, the piece of pepper, 50 g of tomato, the parsley, salt, and pepper. Shape the slab-shaped dough the size of the minced steak and pan fry with 2 tablespoons olive oil 3 minutes on each side.
4. Grill the slice of country bread.
5. Cut the remaining tomato into carpaccio.
6. Arrange half of the tomato carpaccio on the slice of bread, drizzle with olive oil, season with salt, pepper, and basil. Put over the chickpea galette. Finish with the rest of the carpaccio season. Enjoy it immediately.

Nutritional fact

Vegetable bread is a complete balanced dish. It is rich in protein, energy complex carbohydrates (bread, chickpeas), fiber, vitamin C, and anti-oxidant lycopene (tomato). It combines many ingredients of the Mediterranean diet, protectors of the cardiovascular system.

Peach fondant

INGREDIENTS

- 2 pears Conference
- 2 eggs
- 1/4 liter of semi-skimmed milk
- 2 tablespoons maple syrup or 3 teaspoons of sugar
- 1 lemon
- 30 g oat flakes
- 1 vanilla pod
- 2 tablespoons rum
- 2 level tablespoons of flaked almonds

INSTRUCTIONS

1. Spread the vanilla pod under the water, then slice it in half and place it with the milk in a saucepan. Heat to a boil, then turn off the heat and let the vanilla brew.
2. Preheat the oven to 180 ° C.
3. Mix the oatmeal. Remove the vanilla pod from cooled milk and gradually mix milk and oatmeal. Add the maple syrup, the rum, then the 2 beaten egg omelet.
4. Wash the lemon and squeeze it. Wash the pears, cut them in half, remove the fibrous central part and the pips, peel them. Lemon them immediately to avoid blackening them. Arrange the 4 half-pears in a gratin dish. Pour over the milk mixture.
5. Bake for 30 minutes at 180 ° C. Check the cooking with a knife tip.
6. Quickly brown the flaked almonds in a non-stick frying pan and decorate the fondant.

Nutritional fact

Not very sweet, high in fiber with pears and oatmeal, this low-glycemic dessert is suitable for diabetes. Providing only 190 kcal per serving, it can also be consumed in case of overweight.

Exotic fruit verrines

INGREDIENTS

- 2 kiwis
- 1 mango
- 1/2 grenade
- 1/4 liter of semi-skimmed milk
- 2 eggs
- 25 g of sugar
- 1 vanilla pod
- 2 half-sheets of gelatin or 1/2 teaspoon of agar agar

INSTRUCTIONS

1. Wash the vanilla pod, slice it in half, and place it in a saucepan with the milk. Heat and stop the fire just before boiling. Let the vanilla steep in the milk.
2. Position the gelatin in a bowl of cold water.
3. Separate the whites and egg yolks. Whip the yolks with the sugar. Add the cooled and filtered milk. Pour everything into the saucepan and cook on low heat, continually stirring until the cream thickens. Add drained half-leaves of gelatin or agar-agar, wait for their complete dissolution to cut the fire. Divide the custard into four glasses and refrigerate for at least 2 hours.
4. Wash the fruits under running water and sponge them out. Peel the kiwis and mango and cut them into cubes. Collect the grains from the pomegranate. Mix these fruits gently and divide them into the glasses. Enjoy it immediately.

SHORTBREAD WITH JAM

INGREDIENTS

- 100 g of wheat flour type 55
- 50 g butter or margarine rich in omega 3 not lightened
- 50 g of sugar
- 1 egg
- 120 g of strawberry or apricot jam, homemade if possible
- 2 tablespoons icing sugar
- 1 large star-shaped cookie cutter
- 1 round-shaped cookie cutter 1.5 cm in diameter

INSTRUCTIONS

1. Separate the whites from the egg yolk.
2. In a bowl, mix the flour, sugar, and butter until you have a texture of sand. Add the egg yolk to mix the dough ball. Let the dough rest in the refrigerator for at least 30 minutes.
3. Preheat the oven to 180 ° C. Arrange a sheet of baking paper on a baking sheet.
4. Spread the dough. Cut star-shaped shortbread. In half of these shortbreads, cut a small circle of dough in the middle.
5. Arrange the shortbread on the plate and bake for 15 minutes.
6. Let the shortbread a little cool. Cover each shortbread with jam and sprinkle each shortbread with icing sugar. Arrange the shortbreads pierced over jammed biscuits.

Nutritional fact

Made with flour and jam, these biscuits are rich in carbohydrates and energy. They have their place at the end of a meal without starch or snack after a light lunch. They can also be used as a snack, in recovery after a sports training.

Low in fat, they are suitable for hypercholesterolemia.

Chocolate Pear Charlotte

INGREDIENTS

- 18 biscuits with a spoon
- 1 tablespoon liquid vanilla extract
- 2 beautiful ripe pears
- 2 jars of chocolate cream-dessert (250 g)
- 1 lemon
- 1 tablespoon chocolate granules

INSTRUCTIONS

1. Wash the lemon under running water, sponge it, and squeeze it.
2. Wash the pears, peel them, and remove any excessively ripe parts. Cut them into cubes. Place them in a small saucepan with the lemon juice. Cook them covered over low heat for 20 minutes. At the end of cooking, crush them in the sauce.
3. Mix the vanilla extract with 4 tablespoons of water. Dip the biscuits very quickly in the vanilla and line the bottom and edges of 4 ramekins. Spread half of the cooled compote on the biscuits. Pour over the chocolate cream (a 1/2 pot per ramekin). Finish with the remaining compote. Place the charlottes in the refrigerator for at least 4 hours.
4. Unmould the charlottes just before serving and decorate them with chocolate granules.

Nutritional fact

The charlotte pear/chocolate is a dessert or energetic snack rich in carbohydrates. Thanks to the pears, it has good fiber and potassium content.

Very low fat, it is suitable for hypercholesterolemia.

It provides 250 kcal per serving: if you watch your line, take it at the end of a meal without starch.

Poached apricots with blackcurrant

INGREDIENTS

- 2 apricots
- 10 cl of pure blackcurrant juice
- 1 slice of gingerbread
- 1/2 vanilla pod
- 2 teaspoons of aspartame or sucralose powder

INSTRUCTIONS

1. Rinse the vanilla bean under running water and cut in half.
2. Place the blackcurrant juice and vanilla in a small saucepan. Heat until the first tremors, then let the vanilla brew at least 30 minutes.
3. Wash the apricots, pit them, and separate the mumps. Place them in the blackcurrant juice and let them cook for 15 minutes over low heat.
4. At the end of cooking, add the sweetener, remove the vanilla, and then discover the pan so that the blackcurrant juice is reduced.
5. Arrange the slice of gingerbread on a dessert plate. Add the apricot mumps. Sprinkle with blackcurrant syrup.
6. Allow cooling well before eating.

Nutritional fact

Based on apricots and cassis, this dessert is rich in anti-oxidants: beta-carotene (pro-vitamin A) and anthocyanins (dark red pigments) that act synergistically in the body. "Sweet" with a sweetener, it has a reasonable energy intake: 145 kcal per serving.

For a balanced meal, precede your poached apricots with meat, fish, and vegetables (or mixed salad) and dairy.

Bavarian vanilla/coffee

INGREDIENTS

- 1/2 liter of semi-skimmed milk
- 4 egg yolks
- 3 tablespoons of aspartame-based sweetener or sucralose
- 1 vanilla pod
- 2 teaspoons instant coffee
- 4 half-sheets of gelatin
- 1 tablespoon flaked almonds

INSTRUCTIONS

1. Soak 2 half-sheets of gelatin in a bowl of cold water.
2. Heat 1/4 liter of milk with the vanilla pod. When boiling, remove the milk from the heat and let the vanilla brew while it cools.
3. Separate the whites and yolks from 2 eggs.
4. Whisk the yolks, place them in a saucepan and add the cooled milk very gradually. Cook this mixture on low heat, constantly stirring, until the cream coats the spoon. Remove the vanilla bean and add half of the sweetener and the drained gelatin. Whip until the perfect dissolution of the gelatin.
5. Divide the vanilla cream into 4 ramekins and refrigerate for 2 hours.
6. Prepare another coffee cream which you will pour gently into the ramekins and take 2 hours again.
7. Just before serving, quickly pass the almonds in a nonstick skillet for browning and decorating the bavarois.

Nutritional fact

Bavarian is rich in calcium (milk) and protein (milk, egg). Based on semi-skimmed milk and sweetener, its calorie intake is reasonable: 115 kcal per serving. Without sugar, it is suitable for people with diabetes. In case of high cholesterol, consider counting the yolk among your eggs of the week.

CLAFOUTIS MULTI FRUITS

INGREDIENTS

- 400 g (net) of seasonal fruits: peaches, apricots, cherries
- 20 cl of semi-skimmed milk
- 2 eggs
- 40 g flour (2 tablespoons)
- 40 g sugar (2 tablespoons)
- 1 teaspoon liquid vanilla extract

INSTRUCTIONS

1. Wash the fruits under running water. Stake and pit the cherries. Peel the peaches. If the fruit is very ripe, remove any damaged parts. Cut them into small cubes.
2. Preheat the oven to 180 ° C.
3. Beat the omelet eggs and add the sugar. Then gradually add the sifted flour. Finish with milk and vanilla extract.
4. Mix the clafoutis with the fruits. Pour the mixture into an oven pan. Bake for 180 ° C for 30 minutes: check the cooking with a knife tip or a baking needle (the clafoutis is cooked when its dough does not stick to the tip of the knife).

Nutritional fact

Clafoutis multi fruits can take advantage of the good fruit nutrients (except vitamin C degraded by heat): fiber, potassium, beta-carotene, and antioxidant polyphenols. Thanks to eggs and milk, it provides good quality protein and calcium. It is an interesting dessert for children or teenagers who have difficulty eating fruit at the table.

Its energy intake is reasonable: 225 kcal the portion.

LEEK GRATIN

INGREDIENTS

- 2 leeks
- 1 teaspoon of butter
- 1 teaspoon Maïzena
- 12 cl of whole milk
- 50 g grated Emmental cheese
- Nutmeg
- Salt pepper

INSTRUCTIONS

1. Wash the leeks carefully; remove their earthy foot and their green. Cut the whites into pieces and place them in a steamer. Salt them and cook for 25 minutes. Once cooked, let them drain well.
2. Preheat the grill in the oven.
3. Mix the butter and Maïzena. Place them over low heat in a small saucepan to obtain a white roux. Add the milk with a whisk.
4. Add grated nutmeg and half of the Emmental cheese at the end of cooking. Salt lightly and pepper.
5. Arrange the leeks in the bottom of an individual gratin dish. Cover with Mornay sauce and sprinkle with remaining Emmental cheese.

Nutritional fact

- Thanks to milk and Emmental, leek gratin is very rich in calcium: (600 mg per serving, or 50% of the recommended intake for over 50s) and protein of excellent quality.
- Thanks to leeks, it also provides fiber, potassium, and carotenoids with antioxidant properties.
- This dish is particularly adapted to the needs of teenagers, pregnant women, and seniors.

GLUTEN-FREE CHOCOLATE FONDANT

INGREDIENTS

- 100 g of dark chocolate pastry
- 50 g of butter
- 50 g of sugar
- 1 egg
- 40 g of Maïzena
- 1 teaspoon of natural vanilla extract
- 4 individual non-stick molds

INSTRUCTIONS

1. Heat the oven to 180 ° C.
2. Separate the whites from the egg yolk. Add a pinch of salt to the whites and beat in the snow.
3. Cut the chocolate into squares and butter into cubes. Place these two ingredients in a large bowl and microwave in the oven for 1 minute to melt. Mix them well with a whisk.
4. Mix the egg yolk with the sugar. Add the sifted Maïzena, beat well. Then add the chocolate and butter mixture, as well as the vanilla extract. Finally, gently add the white to snow.
5. Divide the dough into the 4 molds — Bake for 10 minutes at 180 ° C.

LIGHT TOMATO PIE

INGREDIENTS

- 4 sheets of brick
- 600 g tomatoes
- 1 beautiful onion
- 1 clove of garlic
- 3 tablespoons of olive oil
- 2 tablespoons of a dry white wine
- 1 bouquet garni
- 1 teaspoon of Provence herbs
- 4 eggs
- 1 mozzarella ball
- Salt pepper

INSTRUCTIONS

1. Peel and slice garlic and onion. Wash the tomatoes under running water, peel them, remove the fibrous core and cut them into wedges.
2. Fry garlic, onion, and tomatoes in 2 tablespoons olive oil. Add the white wine, the bouquet garni, the herbs of Provence, salt, and pepper. Cover, simmer on low heat for 20 minutes. Add some water during cooking if necessary and let reduce at the end of cooking. Take off the bouquet garni.
3. Preheat the thermostat oven 6/7 (200 ° C).
4. Position a sheet of parchment paper in the bottom of a pie plate for four people. Cover with a sheet of brick that you brush with olive oil with a brush. Arrange the other three sheets of brick in the same way.
5. Mix the tomato coulis with the beaten egg omelet. Correct the seasoning if necessary. Arrange this device on the filo paste. Finish with the sliced mozzarella. Bake 15 minutes.

Nutritional fact

The light tomato pie is a complete dish, providing proteins (eggs, mozzarella), complex carbohydrates (brick sheets), fibers and anti-oxidants (tomatoes) simultaneously. Its calorie intake is reasonable: 295 kcal per serving, it is suitable for overweight.

OMELET WITH COTTAGE CHEESE AND FRUITS

INGREDIENT

- 2 eggs
- 1 tbsp. (15 mL) water
- 1/4 cup (60 mL) low-sodium cottage cheese
- 1/2 cup (125 mL) drained canned fruit mingue
- icing sugar (optional)

PREPARATION

1. Whisk eggs and water in a bowl.
2. Spray an 8-inch (20 cm) nonstick skillet with cooking spray. Heat the pan over medium heat. Pour in the egg mixture. As the eggs begin to cook near the wall, using a spatula, gently scrape the cooked portions towards the center. Bend and turn the pan to allow the uncooked egg to flow into the free space.
3. When eggs are cooked on top but still wet, evenly spread the cottage cheese in the center of the omelet. Using a spoon, place a cup of fruit Macedonia on the cheese. Fold each side of the omelet towards the center and the fruit Macedonia.
4. Slide the omelet on a plate. Sprinkle with 1/4 cup of the fruit Macedonia and, if desired, sifted icing sugar.

French toast with apples and mint

Chicken or Vegetarian Curry

This curry is an outstanding low potassium choice and will be high in fibre when eaten with wholemeal rice rather than white rice. You might want to add some extra vegetables, such as green beans (you can even get these frozen). Use a 400 g tin of chickpeas to replace the chicken and enjoy it to turn this dish into a vegetarian option. Bear in mind that both chickpeas and chicken contain phosphate, so if you are prescribed a binder, ensure that you take this dish as directed.

Serves 4

- Twotbsp cooking oil
- 450g chicken in 2.5 cm cubes OR 400g tin of chickpeas
- ½ tsp powdered ginger
- One medium onion
- Twotbsp mango chutney
- 300ml of chicken or vegetable stock
- 150 ml cream
- 55g plain flour (use less is making with Chickpeas e.g. 25g)
- One tsp soft dark brown sugar
- One tsp cayenne pepper (less if you are not keen on a hot curry or omit completely)
- One tsp paprika
- One tsp ground cumin
- Onetbsp turmeric
- One tsp chilli powder
- One tsp ground coriander
- Onetbsp hot curry powder (use mild if you want)

Preparation method

1. Mix the seasoning ingredients in a bowl and add the chickpeas or chicken to coat.
2. In a large heavy saucepan, heat the oil, add the chickpeas or chicken and cook until it is sealed.
3. Add the onion and ginger and cook for another one or two minutes.
4. Add the sugar, chutney, stock, and bring to a boil. Cover and boil for fifteen minutes.
5. Stir in cream and heat, taking care not to boil the sauce.

Serve with boiled rice, preferably vegetables and brown rice.

Chicken and Lemon Casserole

This is a lovely recipe that makes it tasty and economical with cheaper cuts of chicken. The overall potassium content of this dish will be low if cut with rice and boiled low-potassium vegetables such as cabbage, cauliflower, carrots, or green beans.

Serves Four

- Twotbsp honey
- One lemon, zest and juice only, plus one lemon, sliced into thin rounds
- freshly ground black pepper and salt
- 80g (3oz) butter
- 2kg (4lb 4oz) skinless chicken thighs or drumsticks
- Two tsp of dried thyme (optional)
- 500ml hot low salt chicken stock
- Onetbsp of vegetable or olive oil
- Four garlic cloves crushed

Preparation method

1. Preheat the oven to 200°C (180°C Fan)/Gas 6/400°F.
2. Place the lemon zest, lemon juice, and honey into a bowl and whisk until well mixed. Add the chicken pieces and stir until they are fully coated in the mixture. Set aside for ten minutes to marinate.
3. Heat 40g/1½oz of the butter and half of the olive oil in a flame proof casserole pan over a medium heat. Add half of the marinated chicken pieces when the butter is foaming, and fry for five - six minutes, turning periodically, until golden-brown. Put the chicken pieces aside and repeat this process with the remaining chicken pieces and butter oil then set the chicken aside again.
4. Add the lemon slices, garlic cloves, and residual marinade juices to the pan and stir properly, scraping any burned bits off the base of the pan with a wooden spoon. Return the cooked chicken to the pan, add the hot chicken stock and thyme, then stir properly. Take the mixture to the boil, put inside the oven to cook for thirty minutes, or until the chicken is cooked through.
5. Remove the pieces of chicken from the pan and set them aside on a warm plate. Strain the sauce into a saucepan through a fine sieve, using the back of a wooden spoon to press the garlic pulp through the sieve. Simmer the lemon sauce for another five - ten minutes over high heat.
6. Spoon the lemon sauce over the casseroled chicken, then serve.

SIMPLE MEAT DISHES

Pork and Lamb are delicious and versatile meats that can be eaten or even barbequed in basic dishes such as these or as part of a stew. Simply served with mashed or boiled potatoes or for a low potassium option rice or couscous and mixed low potassium vegetables such as broccoli, peas, and carrots.

Minted Lamb Chops

While this recipe preferably calls for fresh herbs, you can make this with any dried herbs you may have in your cupboard; simply reduce the quantity by half.

Serves 2

- Two tbsp fresh mint
- 100g (3½oz) breadcrumbs
- Two lamb chops
- One tbsp fresh parsley
- 100g (3½oz) flour
- Onetbsp of vegetable or olive oil
- One free-range egg, whisked

Preparation method

1. To prepare the lamb chops, mix the mint, parsley and breadcrumbs until well blended. Place into a bowl.
2. Cover the lamb chops in the flour, then dip in the egg and into the breadcrumbs until well coated. Add pepper.
3. Heat a frying pan. Place the lamb chops in the pan and add the oil. Cook for 3 minutes.
4. Turn the chops over and cook for a another 3 minutes.
5. Remove the chops and let them rest for 3 minutes then serve.

Lamb Chops or Honey Glazed Pork

Contrasting flavors from the mustard and honey packs a huge amount of taste in this simple to prepare dish. Try marinating the meat to infuse the flavors into the meat.

Serves 2

- Two lamb or pork chops
- One tsp honey
- 25g (¾oz) butter or low fat spread
- Black pepper
- One tsp wholegrain mustard

Preparation method

1. Spread the butter until creamy.

2. Blend in the mustard and honey. Season with pepper, then mix to a smooth paste
3. Brush the honey mix over your chosen chop, cover and chill for an hour
4. Grill the chops under a hot grill for five minutes each side until cooked. Then serve

Toad in the Hole

Treating yourself to some great quality sausages from the deli or butcher counter will help minimize the amount of additives often added to more processed foods. Adding low potassium flavorings such as mustard is a great way to spice up the sausages.

Serves 4

- ½ tsp English mustard powder
- 100g (3½oz) plain flour
- One egg
- Three thyme sprigs, leaves only (optional)
- 300ml milk
- Two tbsp of vegetable or olive oil
- Eight sausages

Preparation method:

1. Heat the oven to 220°C (200°C Fan)/Gas 7/425°F.
2. Tip the flour and whisk in the mustard powder in a large mixing bowl. In the center, make a well, crack the egg, then pour a dribble of milk in. Stir with a wooden spoon until you have a smooth batter in the well, progressively adding some of the flour. Now add a little more milk and stir until you have mixed both the milk and flour together.
3. Now you should have a smooth, lump-free batter that is the consistency of double cream. Tip it into the jug in which you measured your milk, then stir in the thyme if using, for easier pouring later on.
4. To snip the ties between your sausages, use scissors, then drop them into a 20 x 30 cm roasting tin. Add 1 tablespoon of oil, toss in the sausages to coat the base of the tin thoroughly, then roast in the oven.
5. Remove the hot tray from the oven, then pour in the batter quickly. When it first reaches the hot fat, it should sizzle and bubble a little. Put it back in the oven, then bake for forty minutes until the batter is cooked through, well crisp. If you poke the tip of a knife into the batter in the center of the tray, It should be set, not runny or sticky.

FISH DISHES

Fish is a good source of protein, suitable for substituting any protein lost during dialysis. If cooked with minimum fat, fish is low fat, so if you are trying to lose weight, it is also perfect.

Fish Pie

To make this delicious dish, you can select a mixture of all your favorite fish and it can be made in advance, then either made and frozen for another day or heated up in the microwave.

Serves 4

- 300g (11oz) swede, peeled and cut into smaller pieces
- One tbsp of vegetable or olive oil
- 300g (11oz) potatoes, peeled and cut into smaller pieces
- One tsp dried mixed herbs (or fresh)
- One onion, finely chopped
- 200g (7oz) cream cheese (herbs and garlic flavor)
- 600g (1lb 3oz) fish pie mix, any bones removed
- 20g (½oz) cheddar cheese, finely grated
- Approximately 75ml semi-skimmed milk

Preparation method

1. Cook the swede and potatoes in boiling water.
2. Meanwhile, in a large non-stick frying pan, heat the oil. Add the herbs and onion and cook gently until the onion is tender but not browned.
3. In the frying pan, add the fish and heat until the fish is just cooked. Add the cream cheese and stir over the heat until the cream cheese is melted and nearly boiling hot. Gradually add the milk for a nice creamy sauce. Add pepper
4. Spoon the fish mixture into an ovenproof dish that is pre-warmed. Drain and mash the swede and the hot potatoes. Using the fish mixture to top it up. Sprinkle with grated cheese and place until the cheese has melted and browned under a hot grill. Serve with seasonal vegetables.

Kedgeree

This is a flexible meal that can be served as a main dish, snack or starter.

Serves 4

- ½ onion finely sliced
- 200g (7oz) long grain rice
- One tbsp of vegetable or olive oil
- 400g (14oz) poached smoked haddock or cod filets
- Two teaspoons curry powder
- Four hard boiled eggs
- ½ a lemon
- 400ml low salt chicken stock

Preparation method

1. Warm the oil in a big frying pan, add the onion and fry until softened. To coat the rice in the oil, add the curry powder and rice and stir. Add the water or stock. Cover with a tight fitting lid or tin foil and allow to boil on a low heat until most of the water has been absorbed (about 10 minutes).
2. Place the fish and quartered eggs on top of the rice and replace the lid when most of the water has been absorbed. Continue to cook for another few minutes on the lowest heat and then turn off the heat, leaving the covered rice, fish and eggs to steam for five - ten minutes, allowing the fish to warm through the lid. Remove the lid when after 5 - 10 minutes, and fork the fish with a squeeze of lemon juice into the rice.

Tuna Pasta Bake

This is a perfect recipe for a brisk supper and you may have all the ingredients in the fridge/cupboard already.

Serves 4

- 25g (1oz) olive oil spread or unsalted butter
- 25g (1oz) plain flour
- ½ tsp mustard or mustard powder
- 200g (7oz) cream cheese
- 400ml milk
- Pepper
- Handful of each; sweet corn and pea
- 130g (4½oz) canned tuna, drained and flaked
- ½ onion, peeled, finely chopped
- 60-80g (2-3oz) dried breadcrumbs (shop brought or homemade)
- 160g (5½oz) pasta (such as penne, fusilli, or macaroni), cooked according to packet instructions, drained

Preparation method:

1. Preheat oven to 200°C (180°C Fan)/Gas 6/400°F.
2. Heat the spread or butter in a frying pan over a medium heat. To make a smooth paste, add the flour when the butter is foaming. Continue to cook, stirring vigorously, then pour in 125ml/4½fl oz of milk for another three - four minutes. Whisk the flour and milk mixture to a smooth paste.
3. Add another 125ml/4½fl oz of milk while the mixture is bubbling and whisk until it bubbles and is absorbed into the mixture.
4. Repeat this with the remaining 250ml/9fl oz of milk. Keep whisking and boil until smooth and thick enough for the back of a spoon to cover the sauce. Stir in the cream cheese and remove the pan from the heat. Season with mustard and pepper.
5. Add the tuna, peas, onion, cooked pasta and sweet corn to the cheese sauce and stir until well mixed.
6. In an ovenproof dish, pour the mixture into it. Sprinkle the breadcrumbs over it. Bake for thirty minutes in the oven, or until the breadcrumbs are golden brown and crisp and the sauce bubbling.

Easy Fish Cakes

You can prepare fishcakes from any pre-cooked fish –tuna, tinned salmon, or even smoked mackerel. You can also bake a haddock fillet or salmon in the oven from frozen or fresh.

Serves 2-3

- Two medium potatoes (or sweet potatoes)
- freshly ground black pepper
- 200g (7oz) cooked flaked fish, either a tin of tuna or salmon, or smoked mackerel
- a small lemon juice only
- Onetbsp of olive oil or vegetable
- 100g(3½oz) cream crackers or similar savoury biscuits (or breadcrumbs if you have them)

Optional extras

- Onetbsp chopped chives or parsley
- Two spring onions, chopped
- One tsp wholegrain mustard
- Onetbsp grated cheddar

Preparation method

1. Preheat oven to 220°C (200°C Fan)/Gas 7/425°F.
2. Peel and then boil the potatoes. After twenty - thirty minutes the potatoes should feel soft if not, cook them for a few more minutes, then rinse and leave them to cool.
3. Mash the potato with a masher, clean fingers or fork or.
4. Add the fish and blend thoroughly. Add the lemon, a small amount of pepper and some of the optional extras you like. Have a taste: you can decide to add more lemon or pepper.
5. In a sandwich bag, put the crackers and wrap them in a layers of kitchen paper or clean tea towel. Using a rolling pin, crush the crackers. Pour the cracker crumbs in a plate.
6. Wet your hands a bit and roll the fishcake mixture into tiny balls. You can flatten them into patties, so don't think too much about making perfect balls. You want a thin coating of crumbs all over the fishcakes to make the outside of the fishcakes moist again and drive them into the bowl of crushed crackers.
7. Place the fish cakes on top and pour the oil over the bottom of a baking tray. Turn them all over once, so that each side has a little oil on it.
8. Bake the fishcakes on one side for ten minutes and then turn the fishcakes over for another ten minutes before putting them back in the oven or until the fishcakes are golden brown. Remove from the oven carefully and leave to cool before serving.

SIDE DISHES

Healthy Chips

These chips are lower in potassium because they are parboiled, so good if you adopt a low potassium diet. They are healthier if you use less oil, so the spray oil is perfect if you want to lose weight.

Serves 4

- A small amount of vegetable, spray oil or olive oil
- 908g (2lb) medium sized Maris Piper potatoes

Preparation method

1. Preheat oven to 240°C (220°C Fan)/Gas 9/475°F. Peel the potatoes with a potato peeler, then remove any blemishes. Slice into approx ½in/1cm thick rectangular chips.
2. Bring a big saucepan of salted water to a boil. Add your chips and cook for four minutes. Drain and leave it aside for ten minutes to dry.
3. Put the chips back to the dry saucepan, cover it with a lid and shake the edges of the chips to rough the edges. This roughness is vital to the chips' texture.
4. Lightly grease the olive oil or spray oil on the metal baking tray. Bake in the oven for twenty minutes, turning periodically, until golden brown on all sides. Move the chips to the tray, spray lightly with oil spray or cover lightly with olive oil. Drain on absorbent kitchen paper and serve.

Dauphinoise Potatoes

These garlicky potatoes make a wonderful side dish for any of the meat or poultry dishes. They're really high in calories, so it's best to stop them if you want to lose weight. Parboiling these potatoes helps reduce the amount of potassium in this dish.

Serves 4-6

- One kg (2lb 4oz) potatoes peeled and chopped
- Three - Four cloves garlic
- Freshly ground black pepper
- ½ teaspoon of freshly grated nutmeg (optional) ● 85-100g (4oz) grated cheddar cheese (optional)
- 500ml (17½fl oz) double cream

Preparation method:

1. Preheat oven to 180°C/Gas 4/350°F.
2. Boil the potatoes on the hob for about ten minutes or until they are slightly soft, but firm on the inside.
3. Drain the cooking water and discard it, then allow the potatoes to cool.
4. Cut the potatoes into thin slices after cooling. As you cut them, put the slices in a bowl.
5. Cut the garlic finely or use a garlic press and add it to the potatoes.
6. Season the potatoes with grated nutmeg and ground black pepper.
7. Pour the cream over the potatoes and blend well. Be gentle so as not to turn the potatoes into a mash
8. Put the potato slices into the gratin dish. They're supposed to come below the top of the dish. Using the back of a spoon or the hands, press the potato down so it forms a solid layer. The cream should come below the top layer of the potato.
9. Sprinkle over the grated cheese if using.
10. Put the potatoes in the oven, bake for forty minutes.

PUDDINGS AND CAKES

We all enjoy a sweet treat. If you are trying to lose weight, remember to restrict your portion sizes.

Many of these recipes are high in sugar and you may want to consider reducing the amount of sugar or using a granulated sweetener if you have diabetes. For people with diabetes, it is safer to take small quantities of high-sugar foods with a meal to slow down sugar absorption.

It is good to have something to accompany desserts, but custard is high in phosphate, whether homemade or made with custard powder, so if you are on a phosphate restriction, try these alternatives:

- Cream, clotted, double or single are fine but be careful if you are trying to lose weight.
- Soya ice cream is lower in phosphate than the dairy alternative.
- Low fat/fat free fromagefrais or crémefraîche are lighter alternatives to cream.

Syrup Sponge Pudding

This recipe is great for giving extra calories but has a high sugar content so be careful if you have diabetes. It is however low in both phosphate and potassium. Replace the syrup with Jam for a change.

Serves 4

- 100g (3½oz) caster sugar
- 100g (3½oz) softened unsalted butter
- Two eggs
- Sixtbsp golden syrup
- 100g (3½oz) self-raising flour

Preparation method

1. Cream the sugar and butter together in a food processor or bowl.
2. Add one egg and mix thoroughly with a spoon of flour to prevent curdling. Add other egg and mix well.
3. Measure your syrup into a buttered pudding dish. Spoon the cake mixture on top of the syrup.
4. Fold in the flour.
5. Cover with buttered foil with a fold to enable for expansion.
6. Bake at 200°C (180°C Fan)/Gas 6/400°F/ for forty minutes until a skewer comes out clean.

Rice Pudding

This recipe uses Soya milk instead of cow's milk as this is lower in phosphate but tastes as good. You can add some jam, honey or syrup if you need to gain weight.

Serves 6

- 200g (7oz) pudding rice
- ½ teaspoon salt
- 800ml soya milk (we used unsweetened)
- Four tablespoons sugar
- ¼ teaspoon nutmeg powder (optional)
- ½ teaspoon vanilla extract, or to taste
- ¼ teaspoon cinnamon powder (optional)

Preparation method

1. Add the rice and soya milk to a large pan and stir as you bring to the boil.
2. Reduce the heat once boiled and simmer for twenty minutes or until the rice is soft.
3. Add the vanilla extract, salt, and sugar, then cook for another two minutes, stirring periodically.
4. Pour the rice pudding into dishes and sprinkle cinnamon or with nutmeg.
5. Serve the rice pudding immediately or allow it to cool and serve cold.

Apple Crumble

Apples are not high in potassium and can be used without problem to your crumble or pie. For a low phosphate alternative, serve with cream instead of a low fat crémefraîche or custard.

Serves Four For the crumble

- 175g (6oz) sugar
- 300g (10½oz) plain flour, sieved pinch of salt
- Knob of butter for greasing
- 200g (7oz) unsalted butter, cubed at room temperature

For the filling

- 50g (2oz) sugar
- 450g (1lb) apples, peeled, cored and cut into 1cm/½in pieces
- Onetbsp plain flour
- One pinch of ground cinnamon

Preparation method

1. Preheat oven to 180°C (160°C Fan)/Gas 4/350°F.
2. Place the sugar and flourin a large bowl and mix properly. Take a few cubes of butter,rub into the flour mixture. Continue rubbing until the mixture looks like breadcrumbs.
3. Put the fruit in a bowl and sprinkle over the flour, cinnamon, and sugar. Stir properly being careful not to break the fruit.
4. Butter a 24cm/9in ovenproof dish. Spoon the fruit mixture into the bottom, and sprinkle the crumble mixture on top.
5. Bake in the oven for forty minutes until the fruit mixture bubbling and the crumble is browned.

Lemon Cheesecake

The following recipe is simple to adapt into a fruit cheesecake just by reducing the amount of lemon, then adding any drained tinned fruit on the top. Soft cheeses such as cream cheese are generally low in phosphate, making them suitable for individuals with phosphate restrictions.

Serves Six for the base

- 100g (3½oz) soft unsalted butter
- 200g (7oz) digestive biscuits

For the topping

- One packet cream cheese (a standard packet typically around 200-300g)
- 250g (9oz) icing sugar (sifted)
- One tub single cream (or whipping cream)
- Juice of One lemon

Preparation method:

1. Whizz the biscuits in a food processor until you have fine crumbs, add the butter through the nozzle in tiny chunks while the processor is still working. You should have a damp dough-like consistency.
2. Butter a tin and press the bottom mixture hard into the bottom of the tin and place it in the refrigerator to set.
3. Beat the cream until it is thickened enough to almost retain its shape. Use an electric whisk if you have one to enable you save time.
4. Beat in the packet of cream cheese until the mixture is smooth.
5. Add the sifted lemon juice and icing sugar and beat again a smooth thick consistency is achieved.
6. Pour the topping on the base and spread, put the tin back in the refrigerator until the topping is set. Add fruit as preferred.

Cherry Shortbread

Shortbread is a low phosphate and low potassium treat as well as being relatively simple to make.

Makes approximately twenty shortbread fingers

- 55g (2oz) caster sugar, plus extra to finish
- 125g (4oz) unsalted butter
- Twotbsp glace cherries – chopped (Optional)
- 180g (6oz) plain flour

Preparation method

1. Heat oven to 190°C (170°C Fan)/Gas 5/375°F.
2. Beat the sugar and the butter together until smooth.
3. Add the flour and stir to get a smooth paste.
4. Add the cherries and stir gently to mix.
5. Turn on to a work surface and roll out gently until the paste is 1cm/½in thick.
6. Cut into fingers or roundsand place on a baking tray. Sprinkle caster sugar on it and chill in the fridge for twenty minutes.
7. Bake in the oven until pale golden-brown. Set aside on a wire rack to cool.

Victoria Sponge Cake

Cakes without dried fruit, chocolate, nuts, and coconut are great choices as they are low in phosphate and potassium. Enjoy as a treat!

Serves 10

- 250g (9oz) caster sugar
- 250g (9oz) unsalted butter, well softened
- Four medium eggs
- A splash of milk (if required)
- 50ml double cream
- 250g (9oz) self-raising flour
- Approximately fivetbsp raspberry jam (add less or more for your preferred taste)

Preparation method

1. Grease two 20 cm shallow cake tins, then line them with parchment for baking. Preheat oven to 180°C (160°C Fan)/Gas 4/350°F.
2. In a wide bowl , add the softened butter and sugar and beat until very pale and fluffy. It is likely that this will take about 5-10 minutes. This can be achieved in a free-standing mixer if needed.
3. Add an egg and a big spoon of flour to the mixture and beat again. Until all the eggs are incorporated, repeat this process. Sift the remaining flour in and use a large metal spoon to fold into the mixture.
4. Add a splash of milk if the mixture does not have a dropping consistency (that is, drops easily off a spoon) add a splash of milk.
5. Split the mixture between the 2 tins, smooth the surface and bake in the oven for twenty-five minutes.
6. Once the cakes have been cooked and cooled they can be sandwiched together. W hisk the double cream until soft peaks form. Spread the jam on top of one of the cakes, then spread the whipped cream on the jam. Sit on top of the second cake and sift over the icing sugar for decoration.

Quick and Easy Flapjacks

The oats in flapjacks are high in soluble fibre; however, watch out for all the added sugar. Try adding dried cranberries or glacé cherries for a change.

Makes 12

- 125g (4oz) melted unsalted butter
- 250g (9oz) porridge oats
- 2-3 tbsps golden syrup
- 125g (4oz) brown sugar

Preparation method

1. In a food processor or large bowl, put all the ingredients and mix thoroughly, making sure the oats maintain their texture.
2. Grease a baking tin lightly in all the mixture with butter and spoon.
3. Press into the corners with the back of a spoon so that the mixture is smooth and score the mixture into twelve squares.
4. Place it in the oven and bake 180°C/350°F/Gas 4 for twenty minutes or until golden brown.

Madeira Cake

Plain cakes are low in phosphate and both potassium so enjoy for an afternoon tea!

Serves 6-8

- 175g (6oz) caster sugar
- 250g (9oz) self-raising flour
- 175g (6oz) unsalted butter, at room temperature
- Three eggs
- One lemon, zest only
- 2-3 tbsp milk

Preparation method

1. Pre-heat oven to 180°C/350°F/Gas 4.
2. Grease an 18cm round cake tin, line the base with greaseproof paper and grease it
3. Cream the sugar and butter together in a bowl until fluffy and pale.
4. Beat in the eggs, one at a time and add a tablespoon of the flour with the last egg to prevent the mixture curdling.
5. Sieve the flour and gently fold in, with milk to give a mixture that falls from the spoon. Fold in the lemon zest.
6. Spoon the mixture into the prepared tin and level the top lightly. Bake on the middle shelf of the oven until goldenbrown on top and a skewer inserted into the center comes out clean.

CHRISTMAS RECIPES

Brie and Cranberry Filo Parcels

These cheesy festive morsels will go down a treat, whether you need a delicious starter for your Christmas dinner or some bites to keep party guests going!

The camembert cheeses and brie are much lower than prawns or pate in phosphate, so these also help if you need to limit your phosphate.

Makes: Twelve parcels Ingredients

- 200g brie or camembert cut into
- 200g pack filo pastry

Twelve even pieces

- 50g salted butter, melted
- Baking sheet lined with baking parchment
- 100g cranberry sauce

Preparation Method

1. Preheat oven to 190C
2. Cut filo pastry into thirty-six squares measuring 8cm x 8cm. Cover with a damp tea towel.
3. For each parcel, take three squares of filo, brush each piece with melted butter and arrange on top of each other to form a star. Place one piece of the cheese and a teaspoon of cranberry sauce in the center of the star. Draw the edges of the filo up to form a parcel. Brush with melted butter.
4. Place on prepared baking sheet in preheated oven for six to ten minutes, until golden and crisp.

Salmon and Chive Paté

Ingredients

- 100g soft white cheese spread e.g. Philadelphia
- 200g tin salmon, drained/boned
- 1/4pt (150ml) mayonnaise
- 50g melted margarine
- Two tablespoons lemon juice
- Two tablespoons chopped chives

Preparation Method

1. Blend the soft cream cheese, mayonnaise, salmon, and lemon juice until mixed. Add the melted margarine gradually and mix properly.

2. Stir in the chives. Pour it into ramekins and refrigerate.

In brief

Salt, potassium, and fluid are the most vital considerations. If you are on a fluid restriction, take special care. All drinks (cold, hot, and alcoholic), fruit juices, jellies, soups, ice lollies, and ice cream must be included in your daily allowance.

An average jelly = 150ml

An average portion of soup = 250ml

An average ice cube = 25ml

An average ice cream scoop = 75ml

Avoid salty snacks e.g. crisps, nuts, etc. These will make you more thirsty.

Be careful if you are on a potassium restriction.

Many seasonal drinks and foods are high in potassium and it would be easy to reach a risky intake if care was not taken, especially at social events.

Sausage and Cranberry Stuffing

Chestnut Stuffing is high in phosphate and potassium so try these yummy Cranberry and Sausage Stuffing Balls.

Ingredients

- One onion, finely chopped
- 200g of lean sausage meat
- 25g butter
- One apple, peeled and grated
- ½ tsp mixed spice
- Four sage leaves, finely sliced
- 200g cranberries, roughly chopped

Method

1. Preheat oven to 200C, gas 6, 180C fan. Cook the onion in the butter until soft. Add the breadcrumbs and stir properly so they soak up all the butter. Let the mixture cool. Tip into a bowl with the apple, cranberries, sausage meat, sage and mixed spice.
2. Mix properly, then roll into balls. Cover and chill for up to 24 hours before cooking.
3. Place in a roasting tin and bake for forty minutes until browned all over.
4. Serve and enjoy

Christmas dinner.

Ingredients

- 1/2 tsp black pepper
- 500g Turkey leftovers
- Two medium apples, peeled and chopped
- Threetbsp butter
- One garlic glove, mince
- Three tbspall purpose flour
- Onetbsp curry powder
- One cup low sodium chicken stock
- ½ tbsp. Dried basil
- One cup rice milk, unsweetened • Handful fresh coriander

Method

1. Pre-heat oven over a medium heat.
2. Add basil and curry powder, mix properly and sauté for some minutes
3. Stir in the flour, continue cooking for a minute
4. Add rice milk and chicken stock while stirring well. Remove from heat.
5. Add coriander and turkey leftovers and heat until piping hot.
6. Serve with boiled pilau andboiled green beans or basmatic or plain rice.

Jammy Sponge Tarts

Mince Pies are high in potassium so try these tasty alternatives.

Ingredients

- 100g (4oz) butter, softened
- 200g (7oz) sweet dessert pastry
- Two medium eggs
- 100g (4oz) caster sugar
- 25g (1oz) semolina
- 75g (3oz) self-raising flour, sifted
- Icing sugar, or dusting
- 4tbsp strawberry jam

You will need: A greased bun tin, big enough to hold twelve tarts

Method

1. Preheat oven to 190C, gas 5, 170C fan. Roll out the pastry on floured surface, then cut into 12x7.5cm fluted rounds, re-rolling the trimmings as needed. Line the bun tin, then place in the refrigerator to chill.
2. Beat the caster sugar and butter together until pale and light, to prepare the topping. Beat the eggs gradually, then add in the flour and semolina. Fill the pastry cases with a little jam, then apply the topping. Bake for twenty minutes or until puffed up. Leave the tart for five minutes to cool in the tin. Dust with the icing sugar, then serve.
3. You can serve with cream such as double, single, or clotted.

Christmas Cake

This recipe uses tinned pineapple, cherries, tinned peaches, and mixed peel as a low potassium alternative to dried fruit.

Ingredients

- 200g mixed peel
- 200g Glace cherries, halved
- 100g tinned pineapple, drained and chopped roughly
- Two eggs, beaten
- 100g tinned peaches, drained and chopped roughly
- onetbsp brandy
- 150g self raising flour
- 250g plain flour
- 200g unsalted butter
- 150g caster sugar
- Two tsp mixed spice
- One tsp nutmeg

Method

1. Pre-heat oven to 300°F/150°C/Gas 4.

2. Grease and line a 7in baking tin.

3. Cream butter and sugar until fluffy and light. Sieve the spices and flour together. Add the flour and eggs alternately to the creamed mixture, mixing well after each addition. Stir in the peel, brandy, and fruit. Turn into the tin and cook for threehours.

4. Ice when cool with white icing. Avoid marzipan which is high in phosphate.

Gingerbread Buche de Noel

Christmas pudding and Christmas cake are very high in potassium. Why not try making this delicious low potassium ginger log.

Ingredients

- 50g treacle
- 50g butter, plus extra for greasing
- 2 balls stem ginger finely grated,
- 50g golden syrup
- four large eggs
- plus twotbsp of the syrup
- 100g plain flour
- 100g dark muscovado sugar, plus extra for dusting
- ½ tsp baking powder
- two tsp ground ginger
- For the icing
- ½ tsp ground cinnamon
- 250g icing sugar
- 200g butter, softened
- Three tbsp ginger syrup from the stem ginger jar
- two tsp vanilla extract

Method

1. Heat the oven to 190C/gas 5/170C fan. Grease a 20 x 30cm Swiss roll tin with baking parchment, grease the parchment a little too. Put the butter, stem ginger, treacle, and syrup in a pan, heat and stir to mix, then set aside to cool.
2. Put the sugar and eggs in a bowl and whisk until fluffy, mousse-like and doubled in size, using an electric hand whisk. This will take about ten minutes. Sift over the flour, spices and baking powder and pour the melted butter mixture into the whisked eggs around the sides of the bowl so that it drips down. Fold all together very carefully with a large metal spoon. Pour the mixture into the Swiss roll tin when just combined, and ease it into the corners. Bake for twelve minutes
3. Lay a sheet of baking parchment large enough to match the cake on your work surface and sprinkle with a little sugar while the sponge is cooking. Tip the cake directly onto the parchment until baked. To score a line about 2 cm from one of the shorter ends, use a small serrated knife to make sure you don't cut all the way through. This will assist in having a tight roll. Roll up from this end gently, rolling the parchment among the layers. On a wire rack, leave to cool like this to help set the shape.

4. Put the ingredients in a bowl to make the icing, and whisk until smooth. Transfer to a piping bag fitted with a big round nozzle or use a plastic sandwich bag to create a hole about 1 cm wide by sniping off one corner. Unroll the sponge and sprinkle two teaspoons of ginger syrup on the surface. Pipe over the inside of the roll with a layer of ginger buttercream, then use the paper underneath to help re-roll into a roulade. For a neat finish, slice off both ends. The buchecan be frozen. Defrost at room temperature before proceeding.
5. Place the Buche on a serving board or plate. To build a strong concertina pattern, use the remaining icing to pipe a thick layer over the top of the sponge, zigzagging backwards and forwards. Decorate with white pearl sprinkles. The buche can be stored for up to five days in a sealed container, or it can be frozen for up to 2 months.

Christmas Pudding

Ingredients

- 100g tinned pineapple chunks (drained and rinsed)
- 100g self raising flour
- 100g glace cherries
- 100g mixed peel
- 75g tinned plums (drained and chopped)
- 75g dried cranberries
- 50g vegetable suet
- 50g dark brown sugar
- 50g porridge oats
- Two teaspoons mixed spice
- Two eggs, beaten
- One tbsp brandy

Method

1. Grease a litre (two pint) pudding dish.
2. Mix together the porridge oats, suet, and fruit. Stir in the brandy.
3. Add the flour, spice, and sugar, thenstir in the eggs.
4. Pour the mixture in the pudding bowl, cover with greaseproof paper, securing the string.
5. Cover the greaseproof with foil, securing the string.
6. Steam for four hours over a pan of hot water.
7. Keep in the fridge for up to a week. Steam for another one hour or microwave for ten minutes before serving.
8. Serve with double cream or brandy butter.

Chapter 8

NUTRITION AND CHRONIC KIDNEY DISEASE

Understand your nutrient needs

Committing to a better eating habits is a good start. In order to understand how your diet affects your health. Let's start with an overview of protein, carbohydrates, and fat, and why each is essential to maintain a healthy body when you have kidney disease.

Carbohydrates

The bulk of your daily diet should be carbohydrates, since they are the body's primary source of nutrition. The body continually burns energy, even when at rest. The body requires energy not only for physical activities, but also for a variety of automatic functions, such as breathing and blood circulation. Without energy, your key organs cannot function.

Carbohydrates are categorized into two groups: simple and complex. Fruit is considered a simple carbohydrate and it is packed with energy, fiber and vitamins your body needs. Complex carbohydrates are present in breads, grains and vegetables. These carbs provide vitamins and minerals as well as energy and fiber.

The goal is to choose sources of carbohydrates that do not "empty" calories, i.e. a carbohydrate food that has nutritional value. It is a waste of calories if a food doesn't have nutrients or vitamins that will sustain the body. People with diabetes can think about carbohydrates even more because regulating carbohydrate foods can help to control blood sugar levels.

Protein

Protein develops muscle and repairs tissue. Protein is also used by the body to build antibodies, which are the anti-illness weapons of the body. Other chemicals in the body, such as enzymes and hormones, are produced from protein. Protein can mostly be found in animal sources (beef, pork, chicken, eggs, milk), but it can also be found in plant sources, especially soy products, nuts, and legumes. There are smaller quantities of protein in most vegetables, and fruit is practically free of protein.

Protein is vital for good health, however, in the later stages of chronic kidney disease, your doctor and renal dietitian can prescribe reducing the amount of protein you consume to reduce the stress on your kidneys as well as the accumulation of protein waste in the blood.

Fats

Fat is an essential component in our diets. It helps transport our cells with vitamins such as A, D, E and K. Fat is used to produce hormones such as estrogen and testosterone. Certain dietary fats that have fatty acids are healthy for our skin, make up linings of the body's cells and help with nerve transmission. However, too much fat can lead to weight gain, heart disease and other health issues.

Fats come in 2 categories: saturated and unsaturated. Saturated fats are present in dairy products and meat. These types of fats, particularly LDL (low density lipoprotein) cholesterol associated with heart disease and clogged arteries, may increase cholesterol. The FDA recommends that the number of saturated fats in your diet should be reduced. Unsaturated fats are present in nuts, fish, and specific oils. These types of fats can help reduce cholesterol. Food is often processed so that the unsaturated fat (such as soybean oil) is hydrogenated or partly hydrogenated. This process increases a type of fa*t known as trans fatty acids*. Trans fat, like saturated fat, can increase the level of LDL and total cholesterol. For a balanced diet, the FDA advises the choice of foods low in bothtrans fats and saturated fats.

Potassium, sodium and phosphorus

These three minerals enable the body to function and the kidneys are carefully balanced. Some foods will need to be restricted as CKD progresses, since the kidneys can no longer get rid of excesses of these minerals taken in from the foods consumed. The doctor will order blood tests in order to track the levels of these minerals.

Nutrition for people with CKD

Proper nutrition is extremely essential for individuals with CKD. When blood pressure is elevated, a lower sodium diet can be recommended for patients in the early stages. Major changes in food consumption may not be the main focus of treatment. But this does not mean that you will not be able to take action to be as healthy as you can be. Food is the fuel that we bring into the body. A healthy diet allows our bodies to work effectively. Also, a healthy diet provides us with enough energy to support our level of activity. Too much food contributes to an excess of calories, which are processed as fat and leads to weight gain. Too little calories can lead to weight and loss of muscle.

Your doctor will refer you to a renal dietician if you are in the later stages. Your nutritionist will develop an eating plan to help you remain healthy and prolong the life of your kidneys.

Chapter 9

Common Questions and Answers about the Renal Diet

Adapting to a new diet is a journey that brings about a lot of discoveries and questions about additional changes and options. The Renal Diet is no exception, and while it can be modified to suit custom preferences and tastes, you may have questions about the choices you make and how different foods and drinks affect your kidneys' health.

Question

Is a plant-based diet required to maximize the benefits of a renal diet?

Answer

A vegan diet is not a requirement of the renal diet, though it can be a great benefit if this is your preference. The most important aspect of eating well is to focus on fresh, plant-based foods, as they are easy to digest and contain significant amounts of nutrients. If you choose lean meats as part of your meal plan, be sure to include as many fresh fruits and vegetables as possible and limit the portions of animal protein with each serving, while increasing the amount of fiber and other nutrients.

Question

What happens if I find out that a specific food in my diet is too high in sodium, phosphorus, potassium or protein? Do I have to eliminate it completely, or may I indulge on occasion?

Answer

If your condition is severe, you may want to consult a doctor or specialist before making a firm decision. For most people, the occasional food choice such as a banana, which is high in potassium, is not going to have a negative impact and is often offset with many other health benefits within the renal diet guidelines, if followed closely. For this reason, there should be no adverse effects on your kidneys or health overall. In some cases, a dietitian or doctor may recommend certain foods outside of the renal diet if they notice a significant improvement in your kidneys and/or to treat another ailment that could be related to kidney issues, such as high blood pressure or diabetes.

Question

What happens if I eat too much of the wrong foods and get off track. Is it too late to start the diet over again?

Answer

While it's important to adhere to this diet as much as possible, especially in more severe cases where renal function is low, don't get distracted with making the wrong food choices by switching back immediately. The odd "slip up" is expected, and anyone can make this error from time to time. The most important thing is to keep the basis of your food choices with your kidneys in mind, to avoid future errors and move towards a healthier lifestyle.

Question

Can I drink the occasional soda on the renal diet? Is it acceptable if the soda is sugar-free?

Answer

Drinking soda of any kind should be avoided, as the sugar content is so high (almost 30 grams of sugar in one can!). Artificial sweeteners in sugar-free sodas tend to be unhealthy and may cause unpleasant side effects of their own. If you want to enjoy a carbonated beverage, choose sparkling water with low sodium. Some of these drinks offer natural flavoring with little or no sugar, which makes them an excellent substitute.

Question

Is there a short list of foods to avoid?

Answer

Initially, when you begin this diet, it can be challenging to determine which foods are best to avoid. Unfortunately, while there is no short list, knowing which foods and types of meals to stay away from becomes easier in time. One of the first steps you can take is to avoid salty foods, which are known to be high in sodium and not a good fit for the renal diet. Foods high in protein should be limited as well, especially red meats. Plant-based sources of protein are much better for digestion, and easier on the kidneys. Foods high in phosphorus and potassium will become common once you familiarize yourself with them. In general, a better way to approach this diet is to focus on the foods you can have, as opposed to those you must limit or avoid.

Question

I've been following the renal diet for several months, but there haven't been any significant improvements to my kidneys. Does the renal diet work for everyone or just some people?

Answer

The answer to this question can vary dramatically, depending on the severity of the disease and stage of renal failure. In extreme cases where dialysis is involved, dietary changes may take much longer to have an impact than in situations where kidney disease has not progressed past the early stages and remains relatively easy to manage with diet. Other factors that may impact the variance in success or kidney improvement include the amount of excess weight, as it can take longer for some people to lose extra weight than others, glucose levels, and various stages of heart disease and/or type-2 diabetes. Given the number of variables that may affect your progress on the renal diet, always allow more time and keep a diary or journal to track any changes you notice. It may take longer than you expect, but by consistently following the meal plans and making better choices, you'll definitely see changes.

Question

How do I know if I'm eating too much protein or sodium? How can I avoid eating more phosphorus or potassium than my kidneys can handle, and how do I know when I've had too much?

Answer

Keeping a journal of your food options for meal planning is an ideal way to review your diet. Stay in regular contact with your doctor and share your meal plans, so they know exactly what you are eating on a daily basis. It may seem like a lot of work, but it's worthwhile until you become used to making informed decisions about the foods you eat. Every individual's circumstance is different: some people may have more leniency with the volume of protein and potassium they can consume, while those who use dialysis may need to restrict their choices further to ensure they can get the most out of the renal diet plan.

Question

Does the renal diet guarantee healthy kidneys if it is used as a preventative diet?

Answer

There is no guarantee that your kidneys will always function the same, and this refers to both healthy and impaired organs. Most people don't pay attention to the health of their kidneys until they are diagnosed with a condition, and only then are they faced with the decision to make dietary changes as soon as possible. Taking preventative measures doesn't necessarily require adherence to the renal diet, though aspects of this way of eating can be implemented into your diet to better support your kidneys while they are working well. If you have family or friends with kidney conditions, eating a renal-cautious diet with them and sharing meals is a good way to show your support while helping yourself at the same time.

The best prevention is eating natural, whole foods, and focusing more on plant-based sources of nutrients. Reduce your animal proteins, and ensure you get the nutrients you need in moderation, without consuming too much sodium or protein. There is never a full guarantee that eating a well-balanced diet will prevent kidney disease completely, though it can be a great defense against renal disease and failure.

Question

Can the renal diet heal kidneys completely and restore their function to before they became infected?

Answer

Once damage to the kidneys occurs, it cannot be reversed; however, improvements can be made to ensure further damage is prevented and better function is restored, at least to an extent. For people who suffer from more advanced stages of renal disease, it is most important that the progress of the condition is arrested, so they can live longer and experience a better-quality life. Adhering to a renal diet is one way to ensure the kidneys get a "break" from toxins. Once you reach the stage of dialysis, it is vital to choose your meals as carefully as possible, as this becomes a requirement for the remainder of your life. If dietary and lifestyle changes can be successfully made prior to this stage, the prognosis is excellent, and you can lead a normal, productive life. Now more than ever, as we learn about the importance of kidney health, management of renal disease becomes a chronic condition with fewer complications, as long as you live a healthy lifestyle.

Question

Can medications interfere with the renal diet plan?

Answer

When prescribed a medication, either for your kidneys or another condition, always take the time to read about possible side effects, including food items to avoid. This may include some foods recommended on the renal diet. If in doubt, avoid any specific foods you may encounter reactions with as a result of the medication and consult with a pharmacist or doctor before proceeding. It's always best to avoid potential complications and play it safe before combining a potentially dangerous mix.

Question

Is kidney failure hereditary?

Answer

While there are some predisposed conditions that could lead to a higher chance of kidney disease or infection, there is no evidence to suggest kidney disease or renal failure is, in itself, hereditary. It is a fully preventable condition, and if you know of any kidney disease history in your family, you may be more likely to pay attention to the warning signs, especially early symptoms. Choosing your foods carefully and avoiding overeating and consuming processed foods will help you prevent kidney problems later in life.

Chapter 10: 30 day Meal Plan to Repair the Kidneys Naturally

DAYS	BREAKFAST	LUNCH/DINNER	DESSERTS AND SNACKS
1	Parmesan Zucchini Frittata	Beef Stroganoff Soup	Lemon Squares
2	Texas Toast Casserole	Buffalo Ranch Chicken Soup	Creamy Pineapple Dessert
3	Apple Cinnamon Rings	Paprika Pork Soup	Blackberry Mountain Pie
4	Zucchini Bread	Coffee and Wine Beef Stew	Buttery Lemon Squares
5	Garlic Mayo Bread	Beef Stew	Chocolate Gelatin Mousse
6	Yogurt Bulgur	Bacon Cheeseburger Soup	Blackberry Cream Cheese Pie
7	Chia Pudding	Pork Steaks	Almond Milk Coffee and Chocolate
8	Goat Cheese Omelet	Pork and Veggie Skewers	Cashew Creamed Coffee with Cocoa Nibs
9	Vanilla Scones	Pork with Bamboo Shoots and Cauliflower	Coconut Creamed Coffee with Cinnamon
10	Olive Bread	Crispy Pork Shoulder	Pecan Pancake

11	Yufka Pies	Frittata with Spicy Sausage	Almond Milk Coffee and Blueberry
12	Breakfast Potato Latkes with Spinach	Pork Stir-Fry Chinese-Style with Muenster Cheese	Blueberry muffins
13	Cherry Tomatoes and Feta Fritatta	Slow Cooker Hungarian Goulash	Oven Baked Eggplant Fries
14	Egg White Scramble	Pork and Bell Pepper Quiche	Gluten-free Dark Choco Almond Butter
15	Beet Smoothie	Grilled salsa	Mango Pear Salsa
16	Cinnamon Apple Water	Ground Turkey with Veggies	Upland Cress and Cauliflower Open-Faced Sandwich
17	Apple and Beet Juice Mix	Turkey & Pumpkin Chili	Zucchini Chips
18	Protein Caramel Latte	Cranberry-lime apple spritzer	Carrot Muffin Cake
19	Lime Spinach Smoothie	Chicken tortilla soup	Blueberry baked bread
20	Protein Coconut Smoothie	Grilled Halloumi and Tuna Salad	Herb bread
21	Strong Spinach and Hemp Smoothie	Tuna Fillets with Greens	Oatmeal Berry Muffins
22	Total Almond Smoothie	One-Pot Seafood Stew	Berry Fruit Salad with Yogurt
23	Ultimate Green Mix Smoothie	Easy Parmesan Crusted Tilapia	Ambrosia

24	Chocolate Smoothie	Hearty Chicken Rice Combo	**Apple Bars**
25	Orange Pineapple Shake	Homemade apple sauce	**Egg Custard**
26	Fruit Vanilla Shake	Grilled Chicken	**Chocolate & Coffee Mousse**
27	Almond Milk	Grilled Chicken with Pineapple & Veggies	**Chocolaty Avocado Mousse**
28	Rosemary Watermelon Water	Mediterranean Burrito	**Chocolaty Chia Pudding**
29	Parmesan Zucchini Frittata	Scallop Ceviche	**Carrot Chia Pudding**
30	Texas Toast Casserole	Yeast dinner rolls	**Apple Chia Pudding**

CONCLUSION

A renal diet is one that is low in phosphorous, protein, and sodium. A renal diet also emphasizes the significance of consuming high-quality protein and typically limiting fluids. Every person's body is different, therefore, it is essential that each patient works with a renal dietitian to come up with a diet that is tailored to the patient's needs.

People with impaired kidney function must stick to a renal or kidney diet to minimize the amount of waste in their blood. Blood waste comes from food and liquids that are ingested. When kidney function is impaired, the kidneys do not adequately filter or extract waste. It may adversely affect the electrolyte levels of a patient if waste is left in the blood. It can also help to improve kidney function and delay the development of total kidney failure by adopting a kidney diet.

www.ingramcontent.com/pod-product-compliance
Lightning Source LLC
Chambersburg PA
CBHW080552220526
45466CB00010B/3122